31 DAYS OF prayer
FOR HUMAN TRAFFICKING

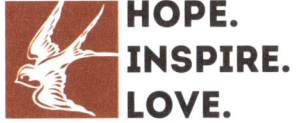

HOPE. INSPIRE. LOVE.

THERE ARE OVER 40 MILLION VICTIMS OF HUMAN TRAFFICKING RIGHT NOW.

We believe the most powerful weapon against human trafficking is prayer. As we stand united and committed in prayer against this heinous and barbaric crime, you are making a difference in the fight for freedom. Because freedom is our legacy!

You Can Be A Prayer Warrior

We invite you to pray over the next 31 days for women, men, and children who are being exploited through trafficking. We need your consistent, intentional, and guided prayers for those rescuing and being rescued will make all the difference. Your prayers are a powerful weapon to shut this perverse industry down. Thank you for coming alongside and praying with fervor, persistence, and effectiveness in the areas of awareness, prevention, protection, strength, guidance, healing, restoration, unity, provision, rescue, and freedom.

Thank you for interceding in prayer on behalf of victims. You are making a difference by bringing hope to the hopeless and a voice to the voiceless. Thank you for joining us as prayer partners and prayer warriors in the fight to end the injustice of human trafficking and modern-day slavery.

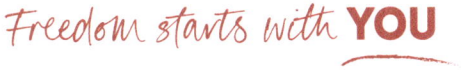

Copyright 2021 Hope Inspire Love, Inc.

All rights reserved. No portion of this prayer guide may be reproduced in any form by any mechanical or electronic means including information storage or retrieval systems, without permission in writing from the copyright owner except for the purposes of research, reviewing or private study according to applicable copyright laws in all territories of distribution.

Inquiries should be addressed to:
Hope Inspire Love, Inc.
P.O. Box 10995
Lancaster, PA 17605
HOPEINSPIRELOVE.ORG/PRAY

31 Days of Prayer for Human Trafficking may be purchased in bulk for educational, church, business, fundraising, or promotinal use. Please visit HopeInspireLove.org/pray for bulk order details.

Scriptures taken from the Holy Bible, New International Version®, NIV®. Copyright © 1973, 1978, 1984, 2011 by Biblica, Inc.™ Used by permission of Zondervan. All rights reserved worldwide. Zondervan.com The "NIV" and "New International Version" are trademarks registered in the United States Patent and Trademark Office by Biblica, Inc.™

Images with people are representative and posed by models.

Printed in the United States of America at ITP of USA, Elizabethtown, PA.

ISBN: 978-0-578-82864-0

STEPS FOR PRAYER

This prayer guide is broken down into 31 prayer themes. Commit to pray for victims of human trafficking for the next thirty-one days. Follow the themes of this prayer guide as you pray for freedom, justice, hope, peace, and healing.

Prepare your heart and mind for prayer:

TIME
Carve out a time for prayer for each day. Remind yourself that you are a child of God, and He wants you to boldly come before His presence.

LOCATION
Find a place where you can be alone and away from distraction. Find a quiet spot where you can turn off the noise of this world and the noise in your head. Turn your cell phone off. Take a Bible, a pen, and this prayer guide.

READ SCRIPTURE
Reset and refocus by reading the listed scripture verses. Each day has one main verse and several additional verses to read. Dive deep into the verses to get your heart ready to enter into a time of prayer.

JOURNAL + NOTES
Pull it all together and reflect. At the end of each prayer time, summarize in the *journal + notes* section some of the things God has spoken to you about. Answer two key questions: "What does that verse and prayer speak to my heart?" and "What shall I do, Lord?"

OPENING PRAYER

Lord, I confess that too many times, I ignore or dismiss or close down my thoughts when I think about or hear about human trafficking. I am busy paying attention to my own life, family, job, ministry, and church and that keeps me from an awareness of the oppressed and marginalized in this prison of living hell. I ask for an awakening of spirit that only You can bring into my mind, my heart, and my spirit.

I take up the plight of those who are trapped in this overwhelming injustice, praying first for safety, next for fortitude, and especially for Your protection. I pray for them to call on Your Name in light of their circumstances and situations…that in hearing their call and cry and love, Your promise in Psalm 91 will be fulfilled: You will rescue; You will protect; You will be with; You will answer; You will deliver; You will honor; and You will show them Your salvation.

Lord, I also ask for myself, that You would challenge me daily to fulfill my unique calling as a carrier of Your Spirit. That I would focus my intercession efforts on those being trafficked, as well as the very institutions and businesses, and parts of society that perpetuate this horror.

Embolden me to individually and collectively proclaim the good news to and for THESE poor, proclaim freedom to and for THESE prisoners; to acknowledge that I need recovery for MY blindness first before I can call out the blindness of OTHERS; and to point out that THESE victims of oppression need freedom. Stir my heart each day as I walk through these thirty-one days of prayer. Wake me with dreams and visions. Burden me with YOUR heart. Change how I think and pray.

PSALM 91

Whoever dwells in the shelter of the Most High will rest in the shadow of the Almighty. I will say of the Lord, "He is my refuge and my fortress, my God, in whom I trust."

Surely he will save you from the fowler's snare and from the deadly pestilence. He will cover you with his feathers, and under his wings you will find refuge; his faithfulness will be your shield and rampart. You will not fear the terror of night, nor the arrow that flies by day, nor the pestilence that stalks in the darkness, nor the plague that destroys at midday. A thousand may fall at your side, ten thousand at your right hand, but it will not come near you. You will only observe with your eyes and see the punishment of the wicked.

If you say, "The Lord is my refuge," and you make the Most High your dwelling, no harm will overtake you, no disaster will come near your tent. For he will command his angels concerning you to guard you in all your ways; they will lift you up in their hands, so that you will not strike your foot against a stone. You will tread on the lion and the cobra; you will trample the great lion and the serpent.

"Because he loves me," says the Lord, "I will rescue him; I will protect him, for he acknowledges my name. He will call on me, and I will answer him; I will be with him in trouble, I will deliver him and honor him. With long life I will satisfy him and show him my salvation."

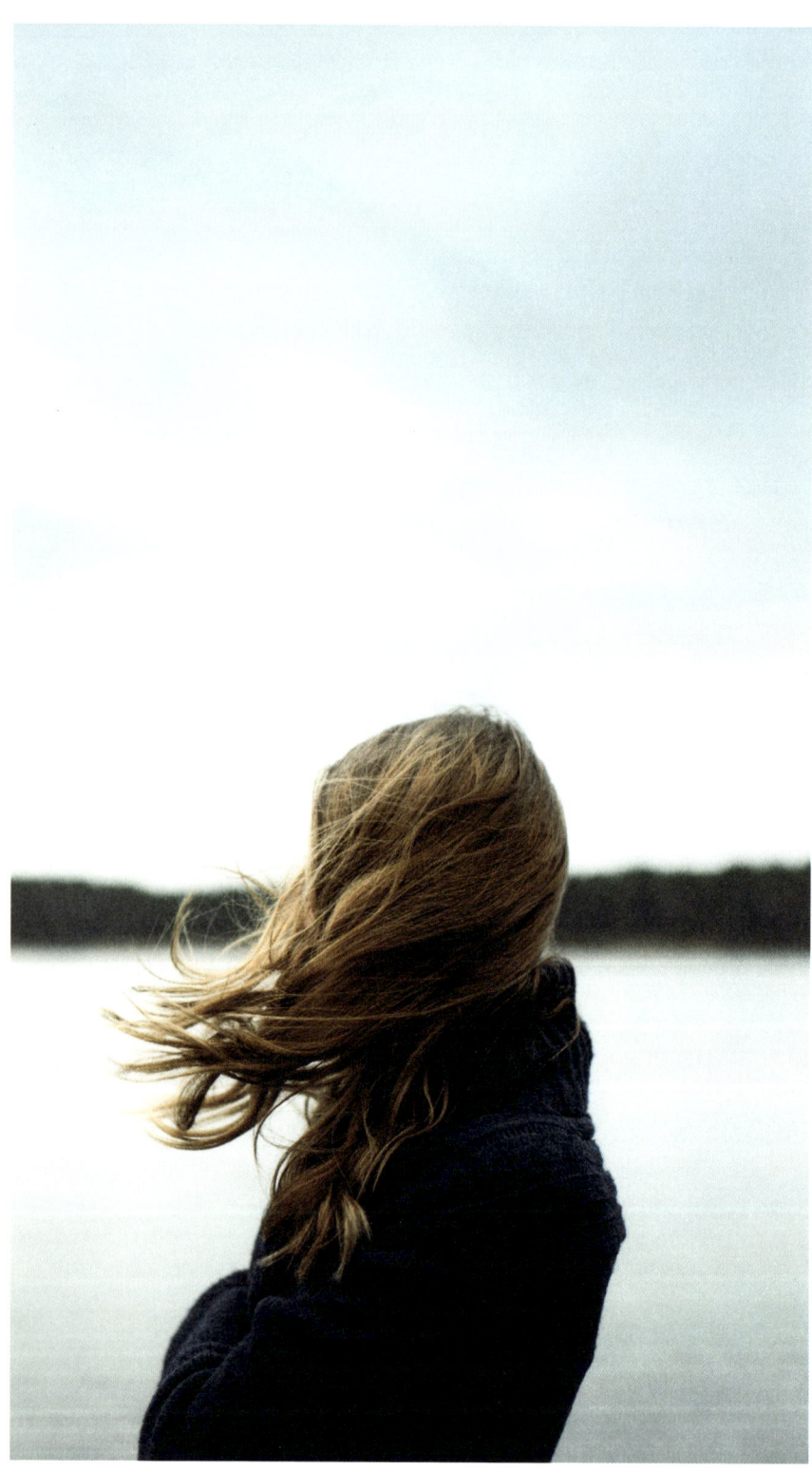

Day 1
PRAY FOR ROOT CAUSES OF HUMAN TRAFFICKING

Father God, I come to You today praying for an understanding of the magnitude and depth of the root causes of human trafficking. Lord, I confess that I only know a small part of what is happening and also have a tendency to "blame the victims" for their plight and circumstances.

I intercede and come against the spiritual forces that cause and grab hold of those that are trapped. In the name of Jesus, I come against untenable circumstances, poverty, oppression from circumstances or by others, lack of human rights, lack of social or economic opportunities, racism, gender inequality, addictions, mental health issues, dangers from conflict or instability in family, lack of self worth and/or self concept, hopelessness, helplessness, and threat of physical violence. For those that are afflicted, suffering, and struggling in this area, I bind their mind to the mind of Christ, and loose every evil spirit that is causing this root problem. I pray that You would intervene in their circumstance and instill hope, provide help, and change their circumstance as only You can. I pray that You are a shield around them, their glory, and the one who lifts their head high. Answer their cries Lord God, sustain them in their time of need. Deliver them! Amen.

Lord, how many are my foes! How many rise up against me! Many are saying of me, "God will not deliver him." But you, Lord, are a shield around me, my glory, the One who lifts my head high. I call out to the Lord, and he answers me from his holy mountain. I lie down and sleep; I wake again, because the Lord sustains me. I will not fear though tens of thousands assail me on every side. Arise, Lord! Deliver me, my God! Strike all my enemies on the jaw; break the teeth of the wicked. From the Lord comes deliverance. May your blessing be on your people.

Psalm 3

OTHER SCRIPTURE VERSES TO READ

Psalm 82: 3-4

journal + notes

31 DAYS OF PRAYER FOR HUMAN TRAFFICKING

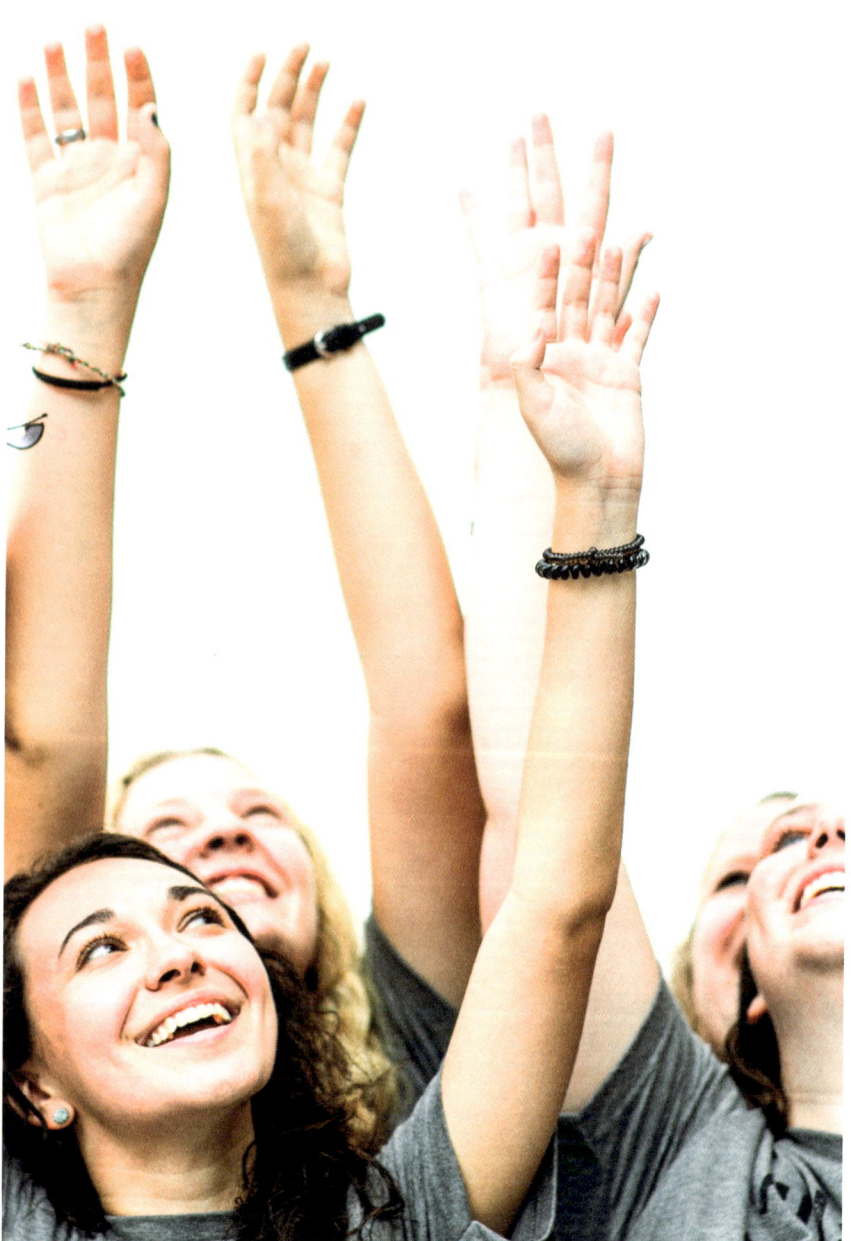

Day 2
PRAY FOR RESCUE AND FREEDOM

Thank You Father, for Your goodness. Thank You that You hear my prayers and that You are near to the hurting. I pray for the liberation of victims who are in bondage of human trafficking and sexual exploitation. You see their hurt. You see their struggle. You hear their prayers, and You hear the prayers that I pray on their behalf.

I know that You desire for each of them to be free, for none to be enslaved, and for all to experience freedom and love. So I come to You now bearing the overwhelming burdens of the enslaved.

Father, hear the cries for help of those lost, hurting, being sold, and abused. Hear their cries for the hope of freedom. I pray that You grant them their prayers and that You move mightily for not one, but for all who are enslaved.

Remove the chains of their oppression. Let the bondage that has become their norm become their past. Provide for them an escape and let them be freed forever. Father, I know the weight of this task is insurmountable in my eyes, but it's not too big for You. I surrender this all to You in Jesus' name, Amen.

Though I walk in the midst of trouble, you preserve my life. You stretch out your hand against the anger of my foes; with your right hand you save me.

Psalm 138:7

OTHER SCRIPTURE VERSES TO READ

Isaiah 58:6, Jeremiah 29:11

journal + notes

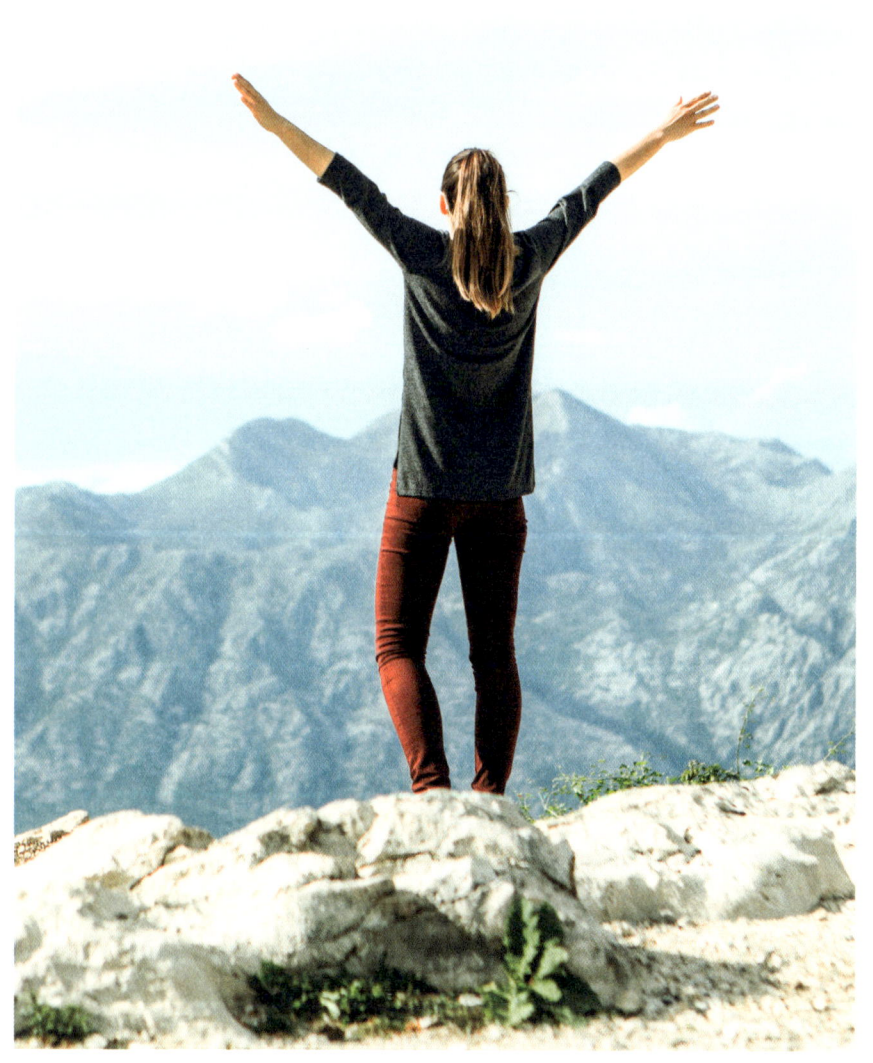

Day 3
PRAY FOR THEIR STRENGTH

Heavenly Father, I come to You today in prayer for victims of human trafficking. They are in need of Your strength. No matter what storms or discouragements they face or how alone they feel, they need Your strength.

In the 23rd Psalm, David acknowledged You as his Shepherd who provided whatever he needed. As David prayed for himself, I pray for the victims that You will help them to "lie down in green pastures" by fully caring for them; lead them by "quiet waters" away from all the noise around them so they may hear Your still, small voice; "restore" their souls because only You can completely renew and restore them by giving them Your strength; guide them in the "paths of righteousness for Your sake" and for Your glory. Even if they "walk through the valley of the shadow of death," help them to know that You are with them.

Today, help them receive all that You have for them and, especially, give them Your strength for this day. Amen!

The Lord is my shepherd, I lack nothing. He makes me lie down in green pastures, he leads me beside quiet waters, he refreshes my soul. He guides me along the right paths for his name's sake. Even though I walk through the darkest valley, I will fear no evil, for you are with me; your rod and your staff, they comfort me. You prepare a table before me in the presence of my enemies. You anoint my head with oil; my cup overflows. Surely your goodness and love will follow me all the days of my life, and I will dwell in the house of the Lord forever.

Psalm 23

OTHER SCRIPTURE VERSES TO READ

Isaiah 40:29, Isaiah 41:10, Nehemiah 8:10, Psalm 46:1-3, 1 Peter 5:10, Philippians 4:13

journal + notes

31 DAYS OF PRAYER FOR HUMAN TRAFFICKING

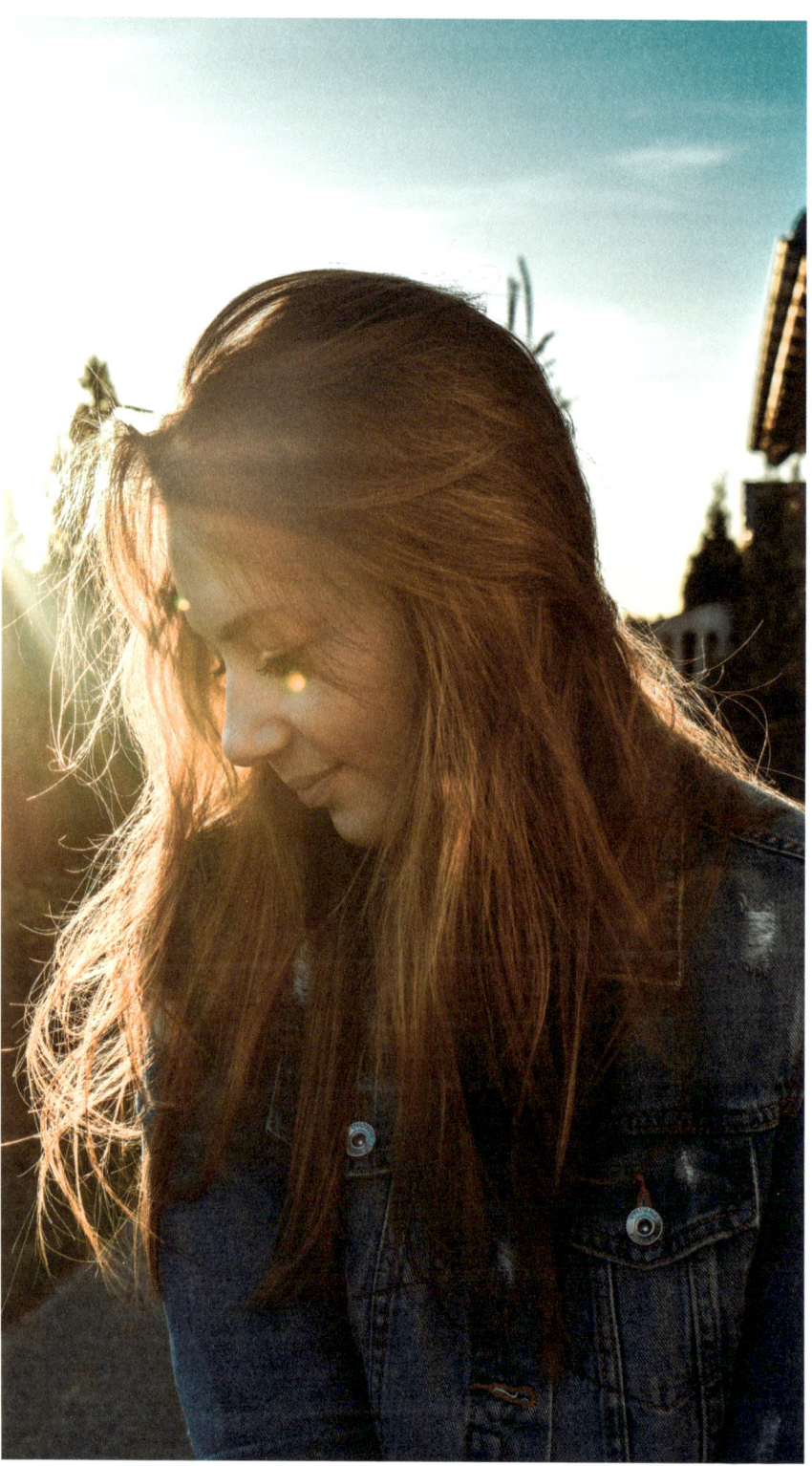

Day 4
PRAY THAT VICTIMS KNOW THEIR WORTH

Sweet Jesus, thank You for creating each one of us in Your image. You created us with such purpose and You, oh Lord, delight in us. I pray that right in this moment, that whoever needs to hear this, that they will know that they are worthy, powerful, brave, relentless, significant, and courageous! Let each sweet spirit see themselves through Your eyes and see the beauty and person as a whole that You have created. You Lord do not make mistakes! Help them find value in themselves over anything of this world.

I pray for those who struggle with low self-esteem and a lack of confidence that they will see themselves the way You see them. You designed them with such intricacy and they have been fearfully and wonderfully made by You. You see them as valuable and worthy regardless of what the world says or they may think. Let them not get caught up in the world's view and need for validation, but find their value in You.

You see them as sons and daughters, and they are more precious than rubies. Let them be confident in their identity through You, Lord. In Your precious name I pray. Amen.

For you created my inmost being; you knit me together in my mother's womb. I praise you because I am fearfully and wonderfully made; your works are wonderful, I know that full well.

Psalm 139:13–14

OTHER SCRIPTURE VERSES TO READ

Isaiah 40:31, Isaiah 64:8, Ephesians 2:10, Song of Songs 4:7, Joshua 1:9, 2 Timothy 1:7, Psalm 28:7, 1 Peter 3:3-4, Proverbs 3:15-18

journal + notes

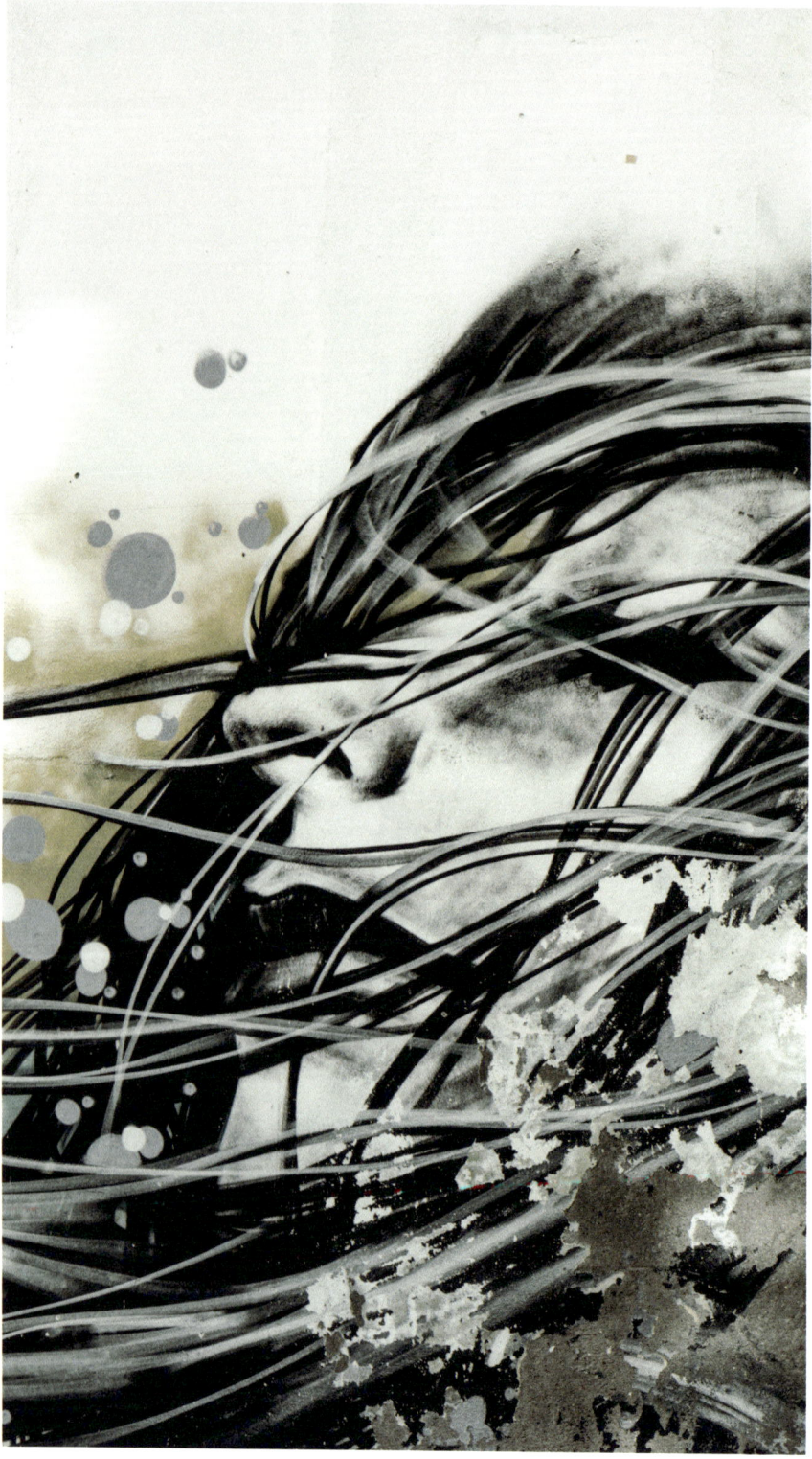

Day 5

PRAY THAT VICTIMS DON'T LOSE THE WILL TO LIVE

Lord Father, I humbly come to You bearing all that is within me. I first give You all the glory and praise because of who You are. Father, I ask You to allow those whose faith and joy was taken from them by the hands of their oppressors, know that You are with them always and that Your love for them is eternal. Increase their spiritual strength, emotions, and mental health. Give them the strength to continue fighting and know that You are by their side.

No matter what the enemy throws at them, let them know that it will never prosper. Remind them of the pain and blood that You endured, and yet You forgave Your abusers. Give them courage to forgive theirs as well. Lord Father, allow them to see that, in You, the true power of love can again flow in their lives. Let them know that You are the true source of joy, and give them favor. Protect them and allow them to live in peace. Give them a new heart that they may love life and begin to enjoy what You have in store for them. Touch their spirit and let them know that no matter where they are, You are with them and that You do not give a spirit of fear. Allow them to continue to fight for the right to live. Amen.

I waited patiently for the Lord; he turned to me and heard my cry. He lifted me out of the slimy pit, out of the mud and mire; he set my feet on a rock and gave me a firm place to stand. He put a new song in my mouth, a hymn of praise to our God. Many will see and fear the Lord and put their trust in him.

Psalm 40:1-3

OTHER SCRIPTURE VERSES TO READ

Jeremiah 30:17, Joshua 1:9, Isaiah 41:10, Jeremiah 29:11, Matthew 11:28, Chronicles 15:7

journal + notes

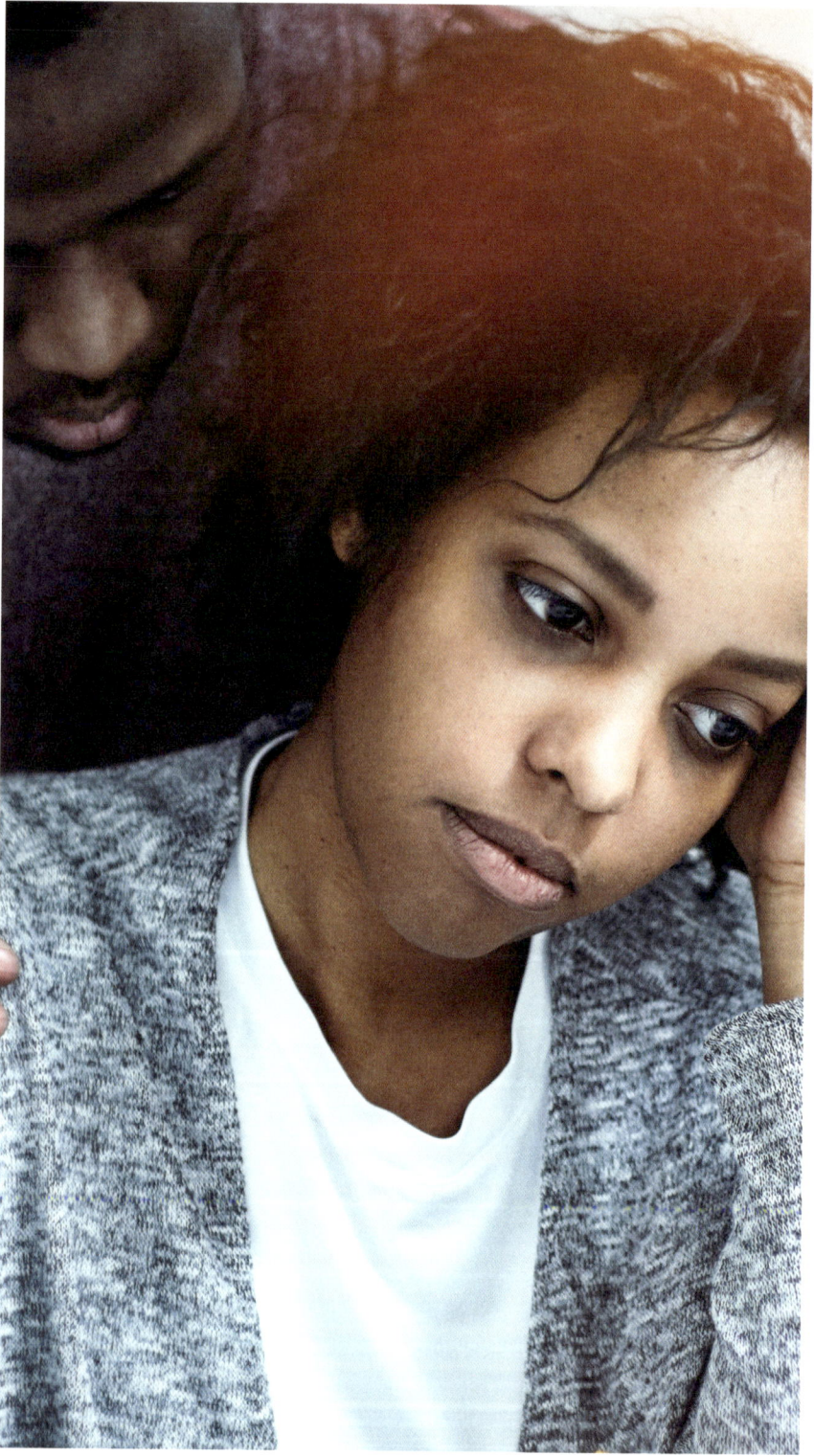

Day 6
PRAY FOR THE FAMILIES OF VICTIMS

Dear Lord, I pray that You will surround the families of victims with Your peace. You are the source of hope and peace. Fill their space with Your presence. Make it so recognizable that they know it can only be You with them. Give their weary hearts rest and cover them with Your love.

I pray that You provide them comfort and that, even in the midst of all the pain and sorrow of this terrible act, You will show Your glory. May Your glory shine, and may the families find comfort in Your presence. Fill them with Your Holy Spirit so that they can find You and a way through the pain. Give them hope. May You bless them and help them in their time of need. Provide them with answers to questions they haven't even thought to ask yet.

I pray that their loved ones will soon be found and rescued and that You will heal their hearts and minds as they heal from trauma and find hope for new life in You. I pray for the families who are hurting and grieving to be comforted by You. I pray for the families and friends of those trafficked that they may receive the grace and strength required to persevere as they agonize over the loss of their missing loved ones, and that You grant them the joy of welcoming them home. Amen.

I keep my eyes always on the Lord. With him at my right hand, I will not be shaken.

Psalm 16:8

OTHER SCRIPTURE VERSES TO READ

Lamentations 3:22-23, Numbers 6:24-26, Colossians 3:13-14, Romans 15:13

journal + notes

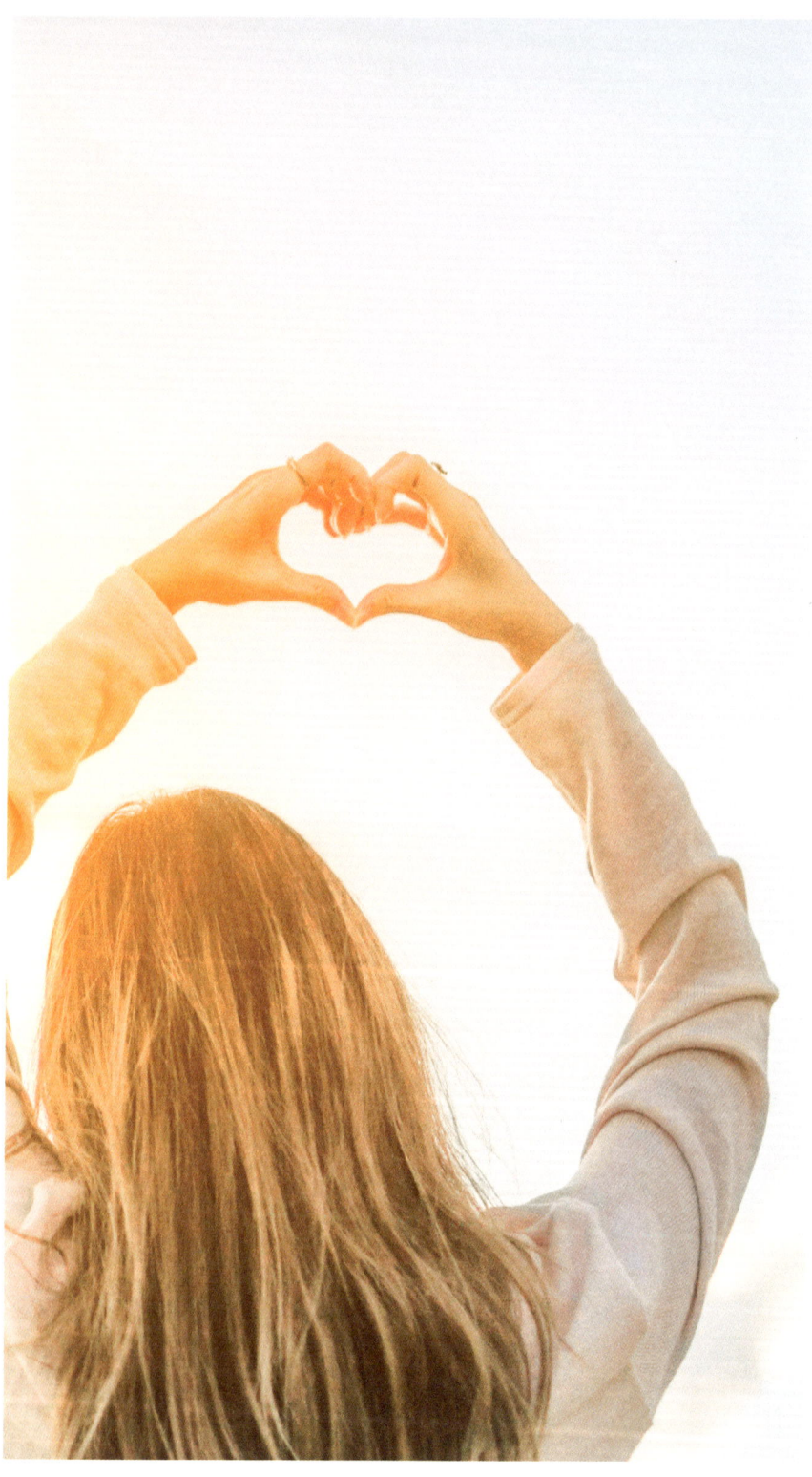

Day 7
PRAY FOR THOSE THAT RESCUE VICTIMS

Father, I come before You today with a heart that begs to be burdened by the very things that burden Your heart. I, Your child and Your Church, want to be so weighted down that it stirs us to action. Allow me to be so unsettled and so deeply offended by the injustices of human trafficking that I cannot just stand by, but I must become a part of the fight. Allow me to become a people who can be trusted, who will take a stand, and who is quick to speak up and speak out. Give me the heart of the Father, a heart of compassion and love, that when I encounter those who have been victimized by human trafficking, they catch a glimpse of how passionately You love them.

Specifically God, I come to You on behalf of those who are currently in this fight. Those who are on the frontlines. I ask for a blanket of protection over them, for boldness and courage, for the spirit of a warrior. I pray for feet that are swift and hands that bring healing. And Father, for those that are still awaiting their rescue, I ask that their day of redemption come quickly, and that until that day comes, You cover them in the shelter of Your wings. Amen.

Vindicate me, my God, and plead my cause against an unfaithful nation. Rescue me from those who are deceitful and wicked.

Psalm 43:1

OTHER SCRIPTURE VERSES TO READ

Psalm 120:2, Psalm 144:11

journal + notes

31 DAYS OF PRAYER FOR HUMAN TRAFFICKING

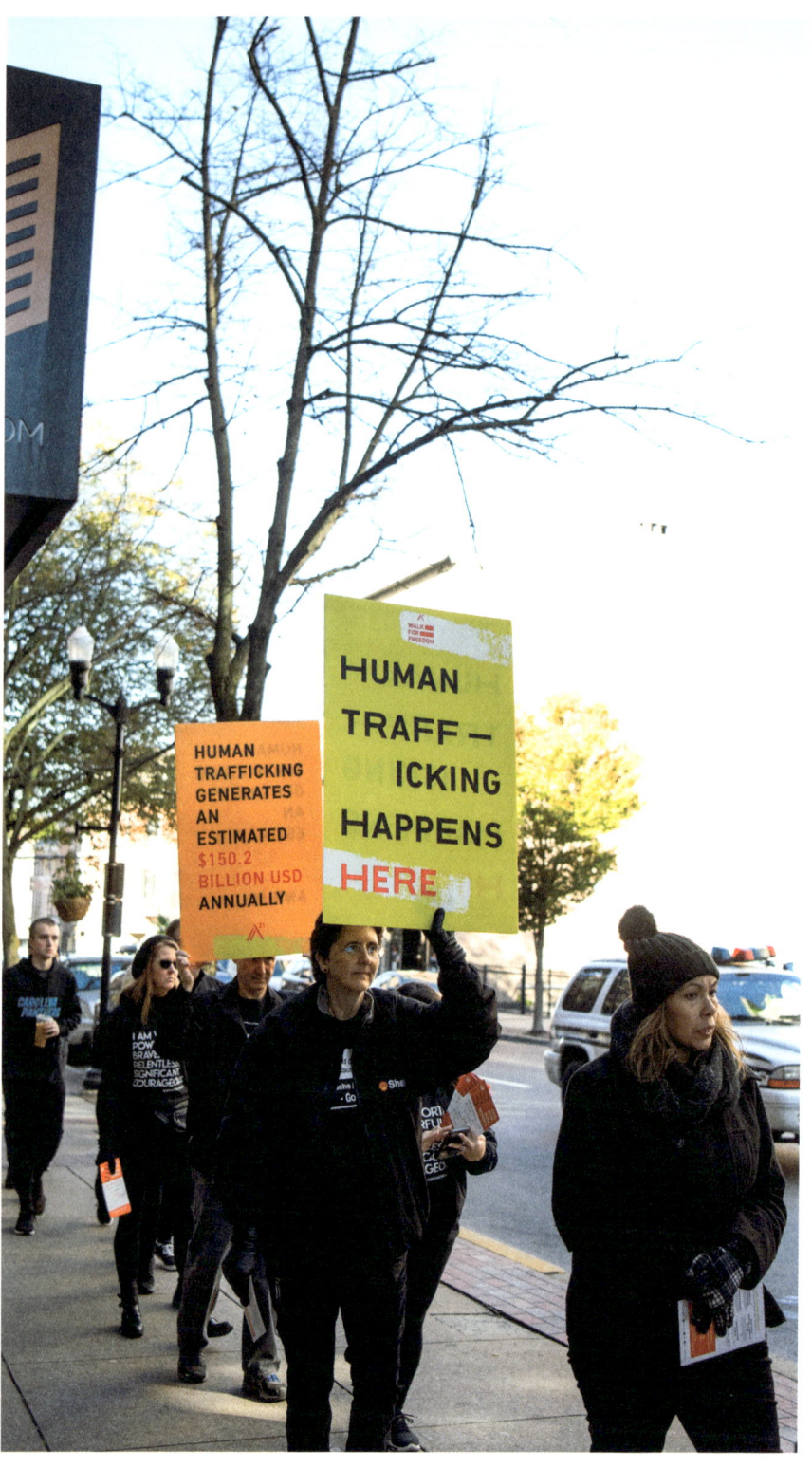

Day 8
PRAY FOR UNIFIED EFFORTS TO RESCUE

Father, I come before Your throne of grace and repent. Forgive me when we don't move as a body, Your Body. Forgive me when I don't walk united, but rather move in self-righteousness and self-preservation. I ask that You give me the humility and strength to lay down my agendas and surrender myself to You. Father, I ask there be no division among us as we do Your work in helping to set the captives free. Thank You that Your Word tells me that two are better than one. I pray I see the fruit of this promise as I unite our efforts to save those trapped in slavery. Thank You that You have created us to live in community. Father, I ask You to bring us together for Your purposes. Raise up a mighty army to rescue victims of human trafficking in our nation and around the world!

Jesus, help me to love like You. Help me to honor my brothers and sisters in anti-human trafficking work, and that together we would be of one heart and mind in going after the ones that desperately need help. I pray that I would come together with such boldness, unity and love, that the world would see You and the freedom that You came to bring. I ask that our efforts would be unified in such a way we see victim after victim rescued and able to start their journey of freedom and restoration. Come, Holy Spirit. I ask all of this in Jesus' name, Amen.

Two are better than one, because they have a good return for their labor.

Ecclesiastes 4:9

OTHER SCRIPTURE VERSES TO READ

Proverbs 27:17, Ephesians 4:32 , 1 Corinthians 1:10, John 13:35 , 3 John 1:8, Romans 15:5, 1 Kings 22:4

journal + notes

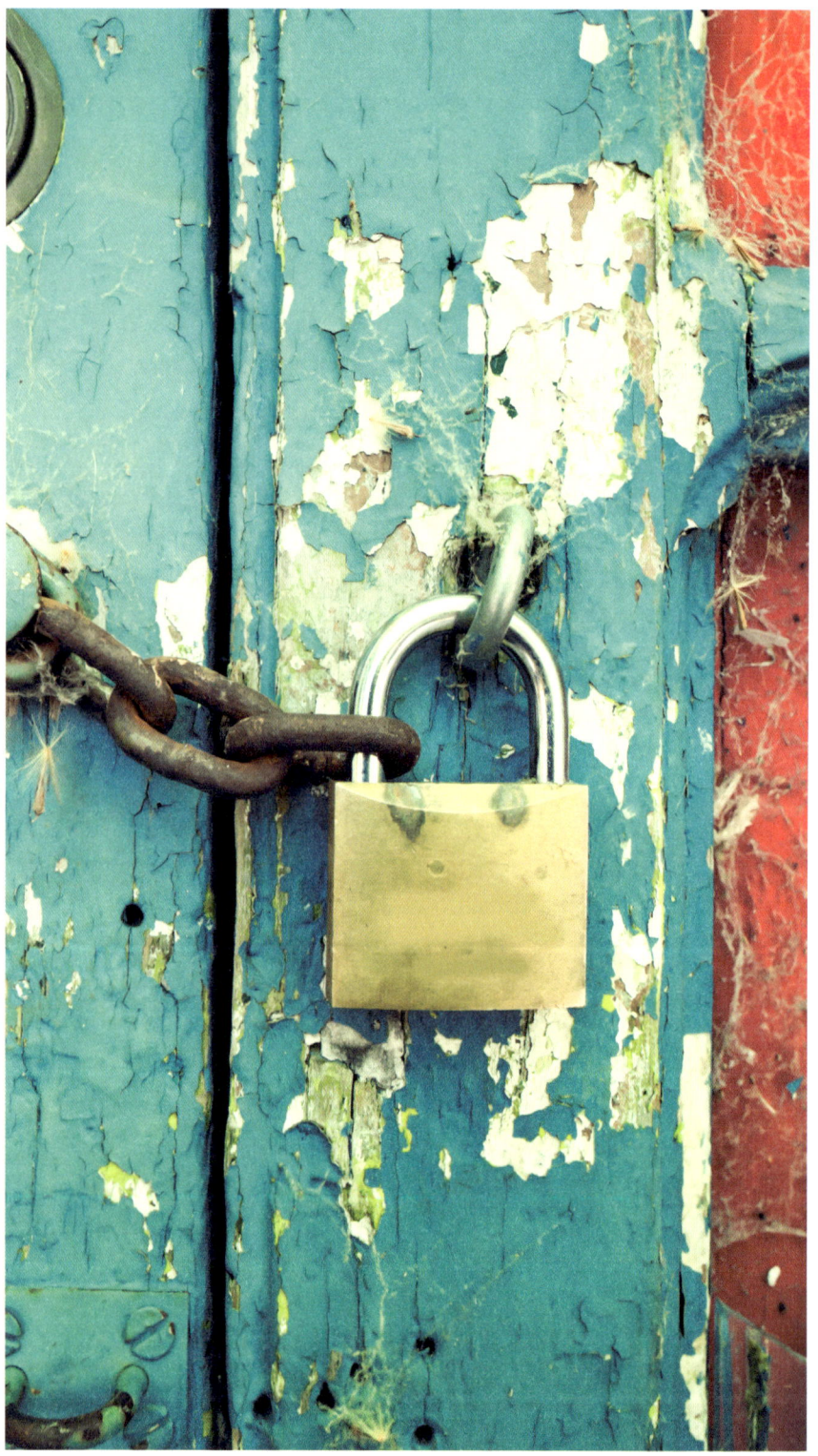

Day 9
PRAY FOR PEOPLE'S EYES TO BE OPENED

Dear Father, as I begin a new day, I would like to take time and lament for those among us that have been desensitized regarding those that have been and are being victimized through human trafficking. I lament that as Paul was blinded in his Damascus road experience and scales prevented him from seeing, that my eyes have also been blinded because of scales of social media, news media, and other forms of communication that have allowed our response to the injustice of human trafficking to diminish.

I pray that the Holy Spirit will ignite a passion within my spirit for the poor, the disenfranchised, and victims taken by force sold or manipulated into human trafficking. I pray that the Holy Spirit will open the eyes of the people and Your servants so that they might respond with fervor the call for justice and response of active engagement toward the eradication of human trafficking in our lifetime…I ask all this in the name of Jesus Christ, Amen.

"Don't be afraid," the prophet answered. "Those who are with us are more than those who are with them." And Elisha prayed, "Open his eyes, Lord, so that he may see." Then the Lord opened the servant's eyes, and he looked and saw the hills full of horses and chariots of fire all around Elisha.

2 Kings 6:16-19

OTHER SCRIPTURE VERSES TO READ

Isaiah 32:3, Acts 26:18, Ephesians 1:18, Isaiah 35:5, 2 Corinthians 4:6, John 14:6

journal + notes

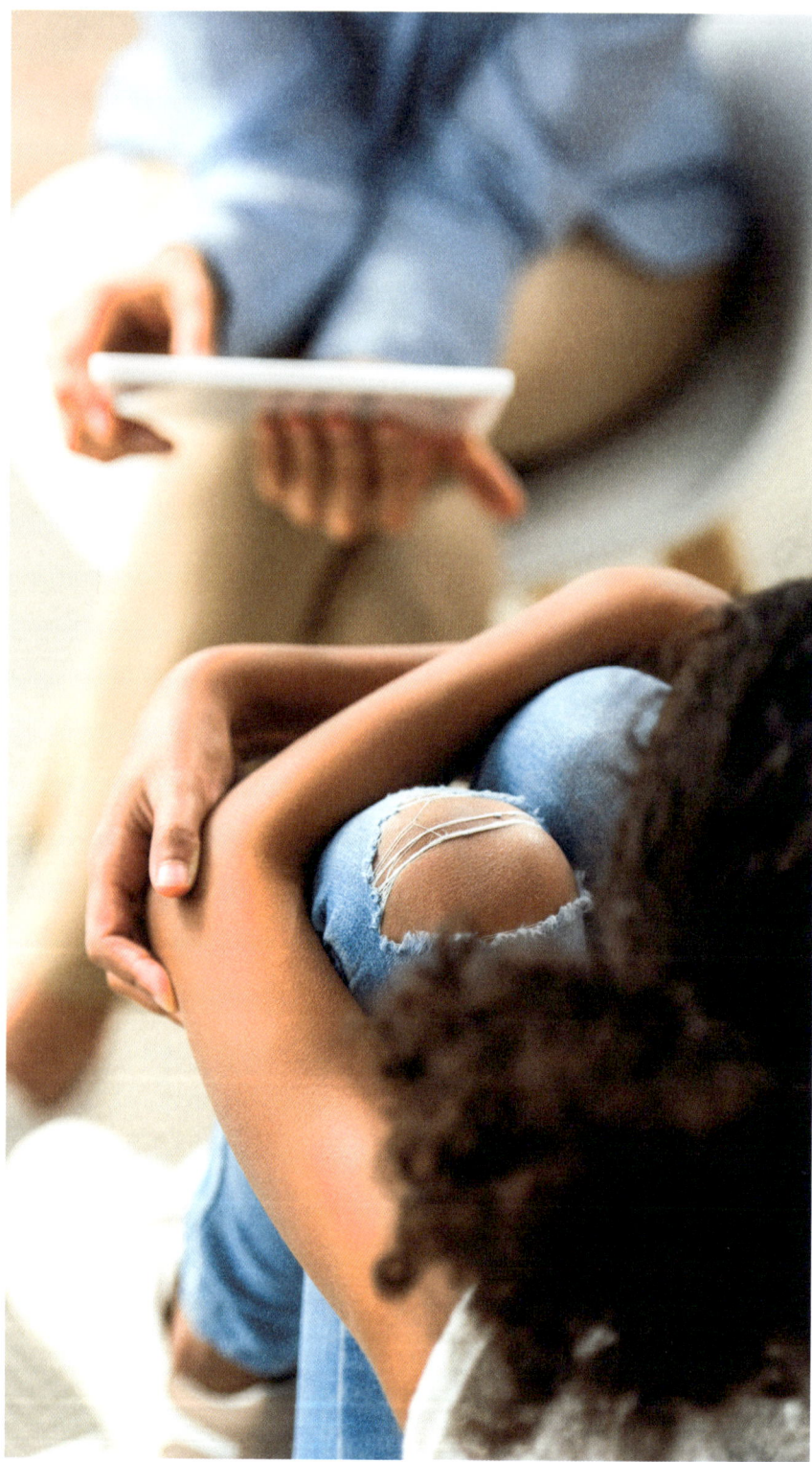

Day 10
PRAY FOR FRONTLINE WARRIORS

Lord, I just want to thank You for all of the frontline warriors: first responders, law enforcement, medical practitioners, counselors, therapists, social workers, lawyers, pastors, restoration coaches, mentors, and countless others in the frontlines of confronting human trafficking. These beautiful souls continue to put their lives on the line to keep all of us and the victims of trafficking safe and healthy. I pray that You will see and honor that commitment.

Lord, I pray that You stand with these frontline warriors and protect them. Protect their hearts and minds, as well as their physical bodies. You know the atrocities that they face each and everyday. Be with them. Honor them. Heal them. God, I pray that You will fill them up with an endurance that surpasses all understanding. You know that burnout is an unfortunate reality within this fight. I pray for a divine rest and refreshment to these individuals, whenever possible, and a Godly relentlessness, whenever on the job. May they be the brightest light in the darkest parts of our communities.

Lord, I pray that Your Holy Spirit guide them daily. I pray that Your Holy Spirit help them discern situations to know where there is trafficking or exploitation going on, so they may act on their behalf. In Your precious name I pray, Amen.

But let all who take refuge in you be glad; let them ever sing for joy. Spread your protection over them, that those who love your name may rejoice in you. Surely, Lord, you bless the righteous; you surround them with your favor as with a shield.

Psalm 5:11–12

OTHER SCRIPTURE VERSES TO READ

Philippians 4:13, 1 Timothy 2:1-2, James 5:16, Philippians 4:19, Numbers 6:24-25, Psalm 46:1-3, Isaiah 41:10

journal + notes

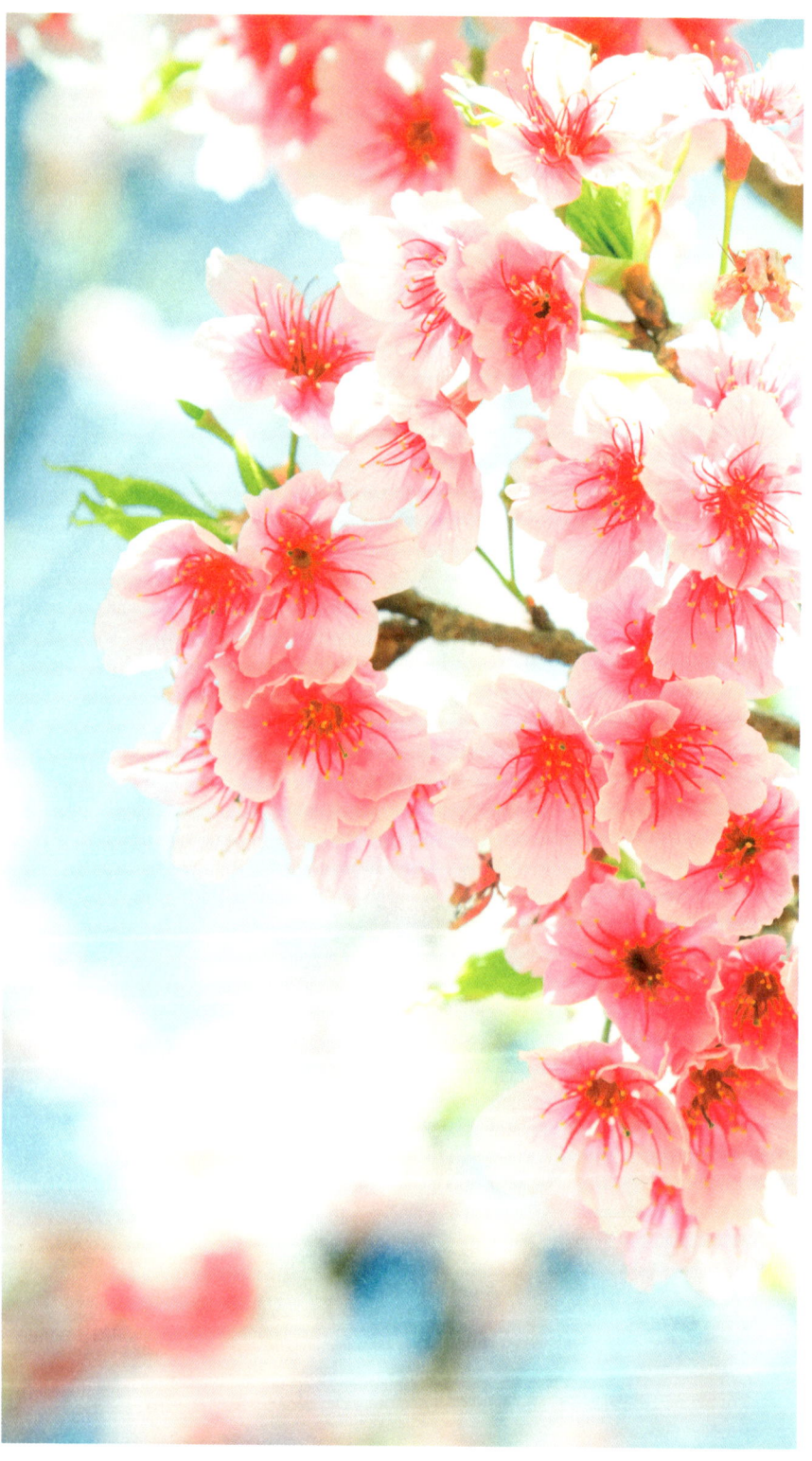

Day 11
PRAY FOR PREVENTION, PROTECTION, AND SAFETY

Father, I come to You in prayer and love for Your protection over our children, youth, and the vulnerable from the evil and selfish greed of human trafficking. May Your people rise up in Your strength, courage, and wisdom to increase awareness and education of this evil reality in our world, nation, and own neighborhoods. Open the hearts and minds of Your people to educate our youth to the lies and deception the enemy uses to draw them into situations disguised as profitable and glamourous. I pray for children to have wisdom to recognize these bad situations before they happen, and the courage to stand firm against those who would have them compromise their convictions.

I pray Your covering of protection and wisdom that no matter where they are, they will not fear or give into temptation. Give Your supernatural strength and courage to those in the horrors of this bondage and slavery for when they cry out in fear and hopelessness, that You make Your presence known to them. May Your hope, Your care, and Your strength be present with them as their "hiding place" to protect them in times of trouble and danger. Father, give me the courage and strength to stand strong and fight for those with no voice and seemingly no hope. In Your powerful name, Amen.

And pray that we may be delivered from wicked and evil people, for not everyone has faith. But the Lord is faithful, and he will strengthen you and protect you from the evil one.

2 Thessalonians 3:2-3

OTHER SCRIPTURE VERSES TO READ

Psalm 34:7-9, 2 Thessalonians 3:3-5, Isaiah 54:17, Isaiah 41:10-12, Psalm 121:7-8, Psalm 32:7

journal + notes

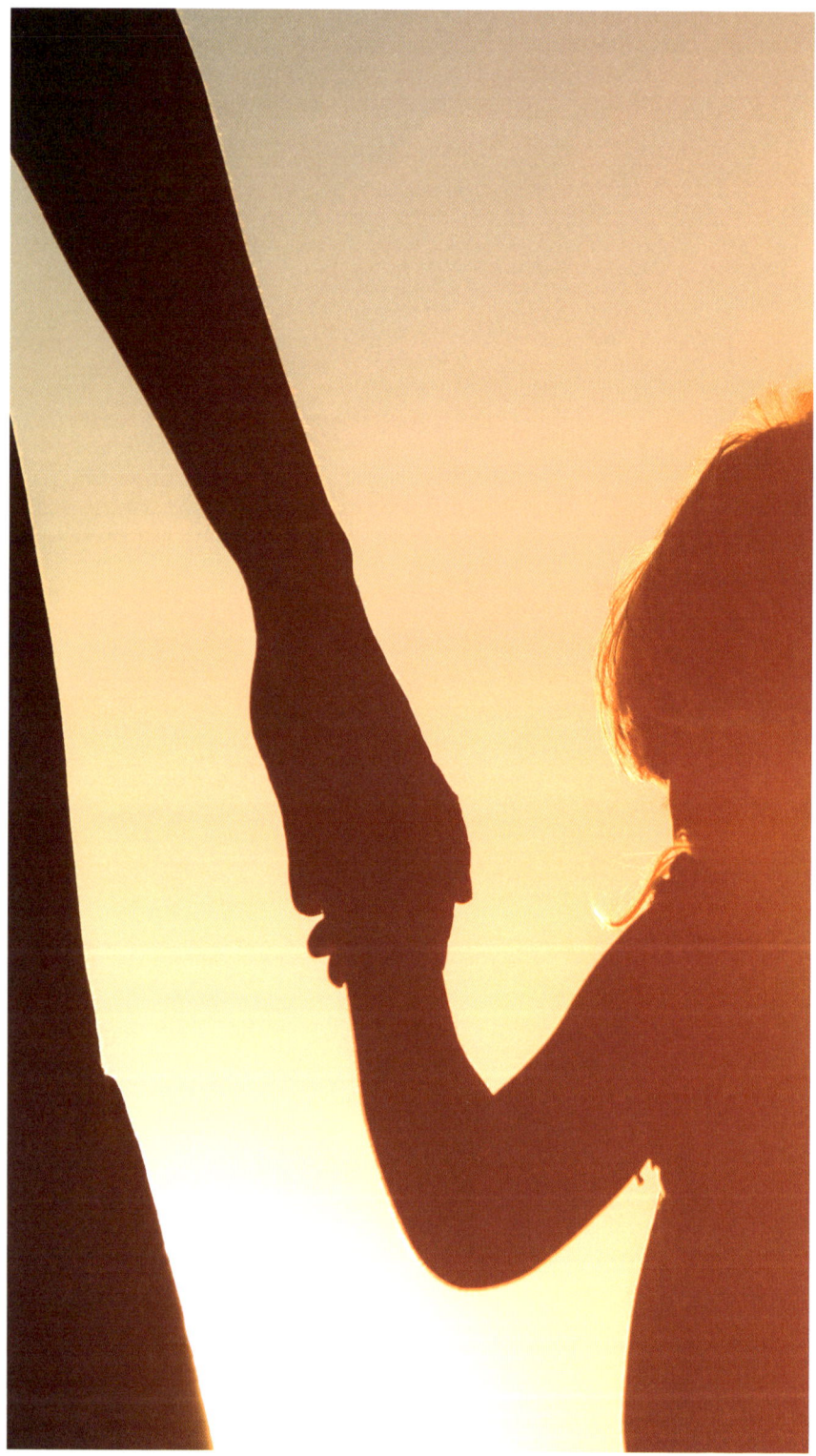

Day 12
PRAY FOR BIOLOGICAL PARENTS, GUARDIANS, AND FOSTER PARENTS

Jesus, thanks for loving me. Your love does not change based on how I act or if I follow You. Help me to allow that love to be my foundation to follow. Father, for each biological parent that doesn't have their baby with them, may they know that all is never lost; that they are loved in ways they can never grasp because they have not seen it. Let them know that You are with them and stand ready to swoop in with grace, mercy, and love that can change everything. Let them know that their relational wounds can be healed and the cycle of pain no longer owns them. Most importantly, be real to them in tangible ways that allow for them to experience the fullness of who You are.

I bring to You each guardian and foster parent. Father, strengthen them for hard days and allow them to experience the joy of the small wins and great days. Remind them that they are caring for others in some of the most real and tangible ways. Give them wisdom to see the acting out and tantrums and grace to parent not the situation but the heart of the child. May they continue to experience an overflow of grace, mercy, and love as they seek to communicate to their children. May community come around them to help shoulder the weight of stepping in to someone's story. Amen.

Be shepherds of God's flock that is under your care, watching over them—not because you must, but because you are willing, as God wants you to be; not pursuing dishonest gain, but eager to serve; not lording it over those entrusted to you, but being examples to the flock.

1 Peter 5:2-3

OTHER SCRIPTURE VERSES TO READ

Philippians 4:6-7, Proverbs 22:6, Psalm 127:3, Deuteronomy 6:6-9, Titus 2:2-8

journal + notes

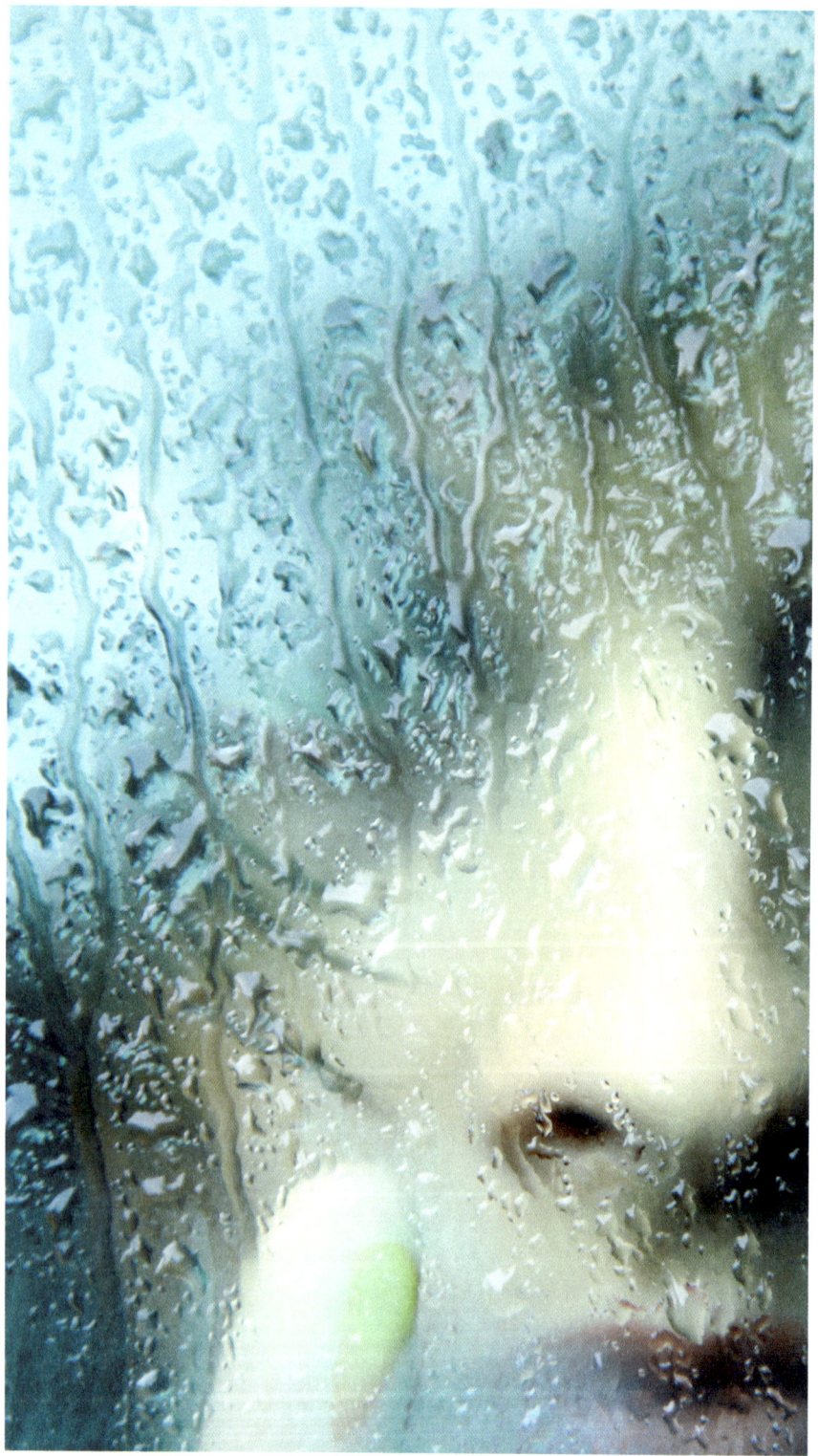

Day 13

PRAY FOR THE REALITY OF TRAFFICKING TO BE UNVEILED

Jesus is the Light of the world and the Light was never given to be hidden. Father, Your Truth is to be set upon a lampstand to dispel the darkness of this age. I pray that the perfect, revealing light of God will leave nothing in the dark. Nothing hidden, nothing beyond the reach of Your light of exposure.

The darkness is as light to You and with confidence, I pray that the ugly, ravaging, life-stealing, dream-killing, joy-snuffing reality of this plague will be unveiled. From the highest offices of power to the cesspools of existence, may Your perfect love shine a revealing light and leave no stone unturned as You deliver justice. I pray that every individual, cell, or group putting their hand to the machine of human trafficking would be exposed in Jesus' name.

I cry out for everyone's eyes to be open to the reality of human trafficking and for a great awareness that would take root in this land resulting in a devastating and demolishing blow to this epidemic. You have given me power and authority through Jesus Christ, and it is in this authority I boldly proclaim freedom from the darkness.

Prayer continues on the next page.

Continued prayer from previous page.

I know that in Your perfect light, there are no shadows, no crevises where evil could reside so as Holy Spirit gives me sight to see into what Your light has exposed, may my awareness increase and my actions be established to war against every form of human trafficking.

May the Church gain next-step clarity against this injustice, for once we know the Truth, freedom will be reality for all. As a church, we do not relent.

In the powerful name of Jesus, I pray, Amen

For whatever is hidden is meant to be disclosed, and whatever is concealed is meant to be brought out into the open.

Mark 4:22

OTHER SCRIPTURE VERSES TO READ

John 8:32, Hebrews 4:12, John 16:13, Psalm 25:5, Luke 12:2, Ephesians 5:11-13, Luke 8:17

journal + notes

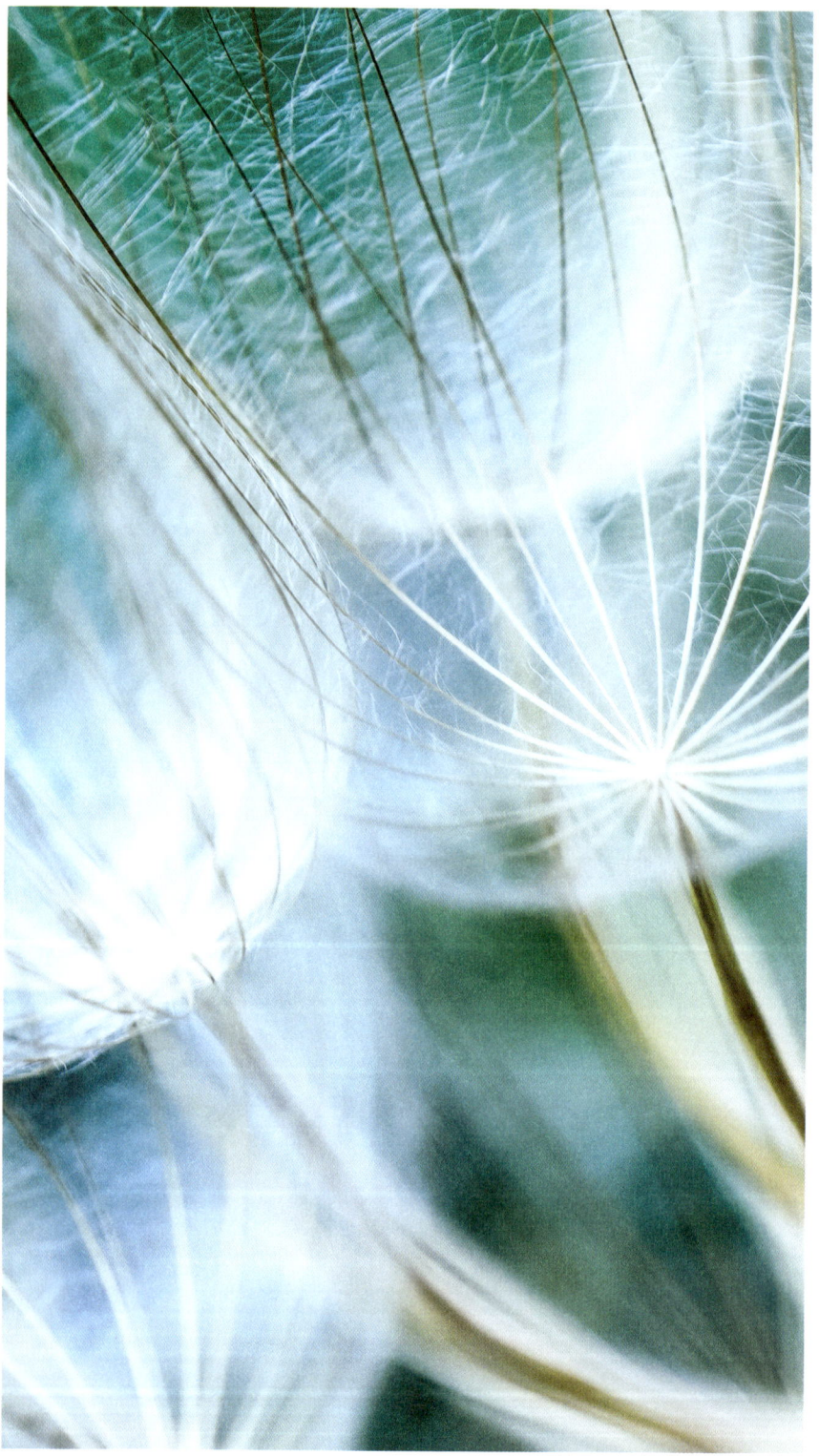

Day 14
PRAY FOR STRATEGIES TO RAISE AWARENESS

God, I thank You that You are the God of wisdom and creativity. I ask for both wisdom and creativity as individuals and organizations create strategies to raise awareness about human trafficking. I ask You to go before these strategies and prepare people's hearts and minds to respond to these efforts. Please open ears and open hearts through these innovative strategies.

I thank You for the many ideas You are planting in us now and ask that for each idea, You give us efficient and prudent action plans for these ideas to awaken people to Your heart for the freedom of these people.

I pray that You guide the work of creating and distributing educational materials, curriculum, books and guides, flyers, trainings, workshops, webinars, galas, print and digital tools, and resources. I also pray that You touch and bless the hearts of those receiving those materials.

Thank You God for Your plans and purposes for our anti-human trafficking efforts, and I ask that You would help me to be attentive to Your voice and guidance in our planning. We also ask that You bring our plans to fruition and that our efforts would be multiplied by You! Amen.

Commit to the Lord whatever you do, and he will establish your plans.

Proverbs 16:3

OTHER SCRIPTURE VERSES TO READ

Proverbs 21:5, Habakkuk 2:2-3, Philippians 4:6, Proverbs 15:22, Proverbs 24:6-8, Philippians 1:6

journal + notes

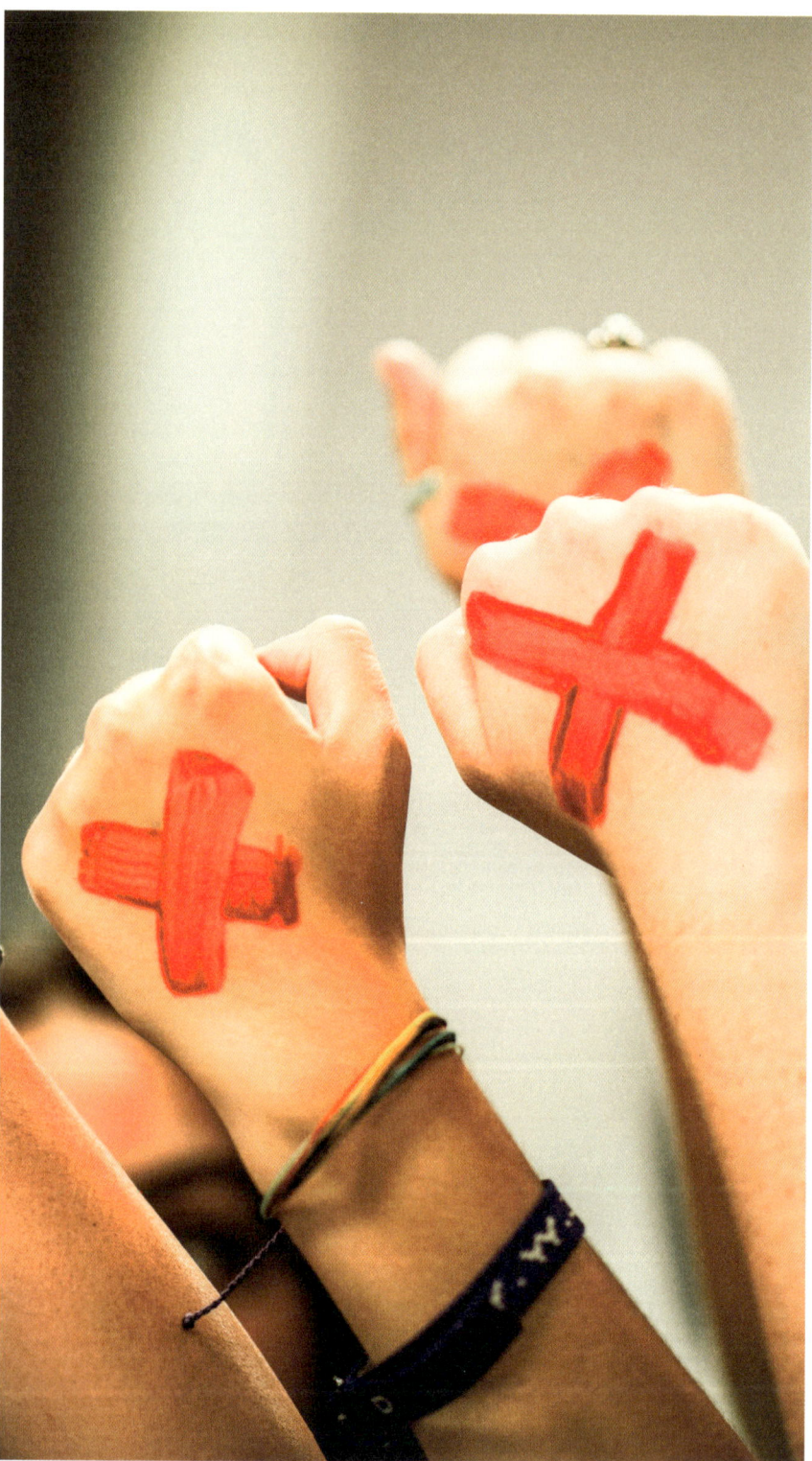

Day 15
PRAY FOR PEOPLE TO BE STIRRED TO ACTION

God, as I think about the awful injustice of human trafficking, it angers my soul and almost paralyzes me with sadness. Lord, as I have these big feelings about Your precious children, please help me to not stay idle in this space. God, use me in a way that will be Your hands and feet to save these precious children of Yours who have no voice right now. Your word says that You have a beautiful plan for each one of us, and I am praying You will show me how I can help these children where someone has tried to take that plan away from them. You have the ultimate and final say in that, and I am believing that I can play a part in helping these victims find what that plan is for them; plans to prosper and not harm them. Sometimes, this all seems so much bigger than me, and I have no idea where to start, and so I do nothing. Help me to do something.

If it means learning more about the signs and warnings, help me to be a good student. If it means helping others learn what to look for and how to assist, help me to be a good teacher. If it means donating to nonprofits that help eradicate human trafficking, help me to give more generously than ever before. If it means coming alongside a victim so they can find hope and peace, give me that opportunity. If it means speaking up when I know something just isn't right, help me to be even more brave. Whatever

Prayer continues on the next page.

Continued prayer from previous page.

You are calling me to do in order to move into action, help me to do it. Intentions aren't good enough, and I'm tired of just sitting around. Help me to be confident that I can partner with You, and You will lead me into making this difference. I may feel inferior, but with Your help, I can do this. No more just talking about it. I'm ready to move into action as part of Your army—willing to go where You send me. I trust You, and I love You, Amen!

"Is not this the kind of fasting I have chosen: to loose the chains of injustice and untie the cords of the yoke, to set the oppressed free and break every yoke? Is it not to share your food with the hungry and to provide the poor wanderer with shelter—when you see the naked, to clothe them, and not to turn away from your own flesh and blood?"

Isaiah 58:6-7

OTHER SCRIPTURE VERSES TO READ

Ezra 1:1, Numbers 11:17, John 16:15, Jeremiah 29:11, Psalms 119:147, James 1:22, James 2:16-17

journal + notes

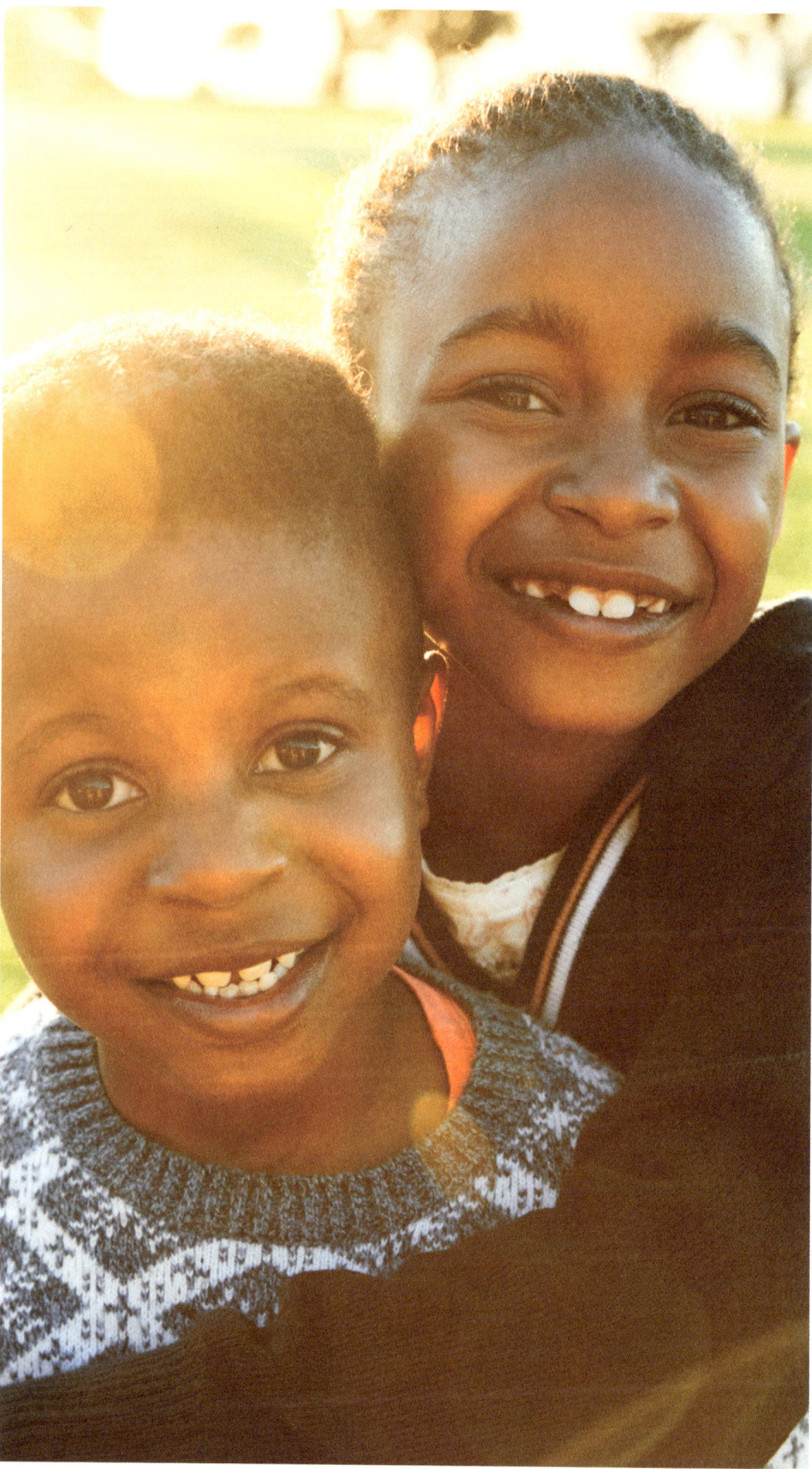

Day 16
PRAY FOR THE PROTECTION OF SONS AND DAUGHTERS

Oh Father, I praise You for You are the Almighty. You are the one from whom all blessings flow. I come before You and plead the blood of Jesus Christ over the precious sons and daughters represented in this predatory industry. God, I know that You are good. And I trust that You have a plan and a purpose for each and every person. Abba Father, in Isaiah 41:10, it is written " Do not fear, for I am with you; do not be dismayed, for I am your God. I will strengthen you and help you; I will uphold you with my righteous right hand."

Children are a precious gift from God. I pray for their protection and safety. I pray for an end to all harm against children who are trapped in this nightmare. I pray for supernatural protection from those who prey upon their vulnerabilities to exploit them.

Strengthen and uphold every son and daughter that is being exploited. I pray that You watch over every single child. Give Your angels charge over them in their coming and going. Rescue and preserve them from all sin and temptations. Sanctify their hearts, oh God. Shelter them in every storm. Defend them in every battle and destroy every mountain in their way. In Your righteous and holy name I pray, Amen.

So do not fear, for I am with you; do not be dismayed, for I am your God. I will strengthen you and help you; I will uphold you with my righteous right hand.

Isaiah 41:10

OTHER SCRIPTURE VERSES TO READ

Psalm 9:9, 2 Thessalonians 3:3, Deuteronomy 31:6, Proverbs 4:6, Psalm 5:11, Proverbs 2:11

journal + notes

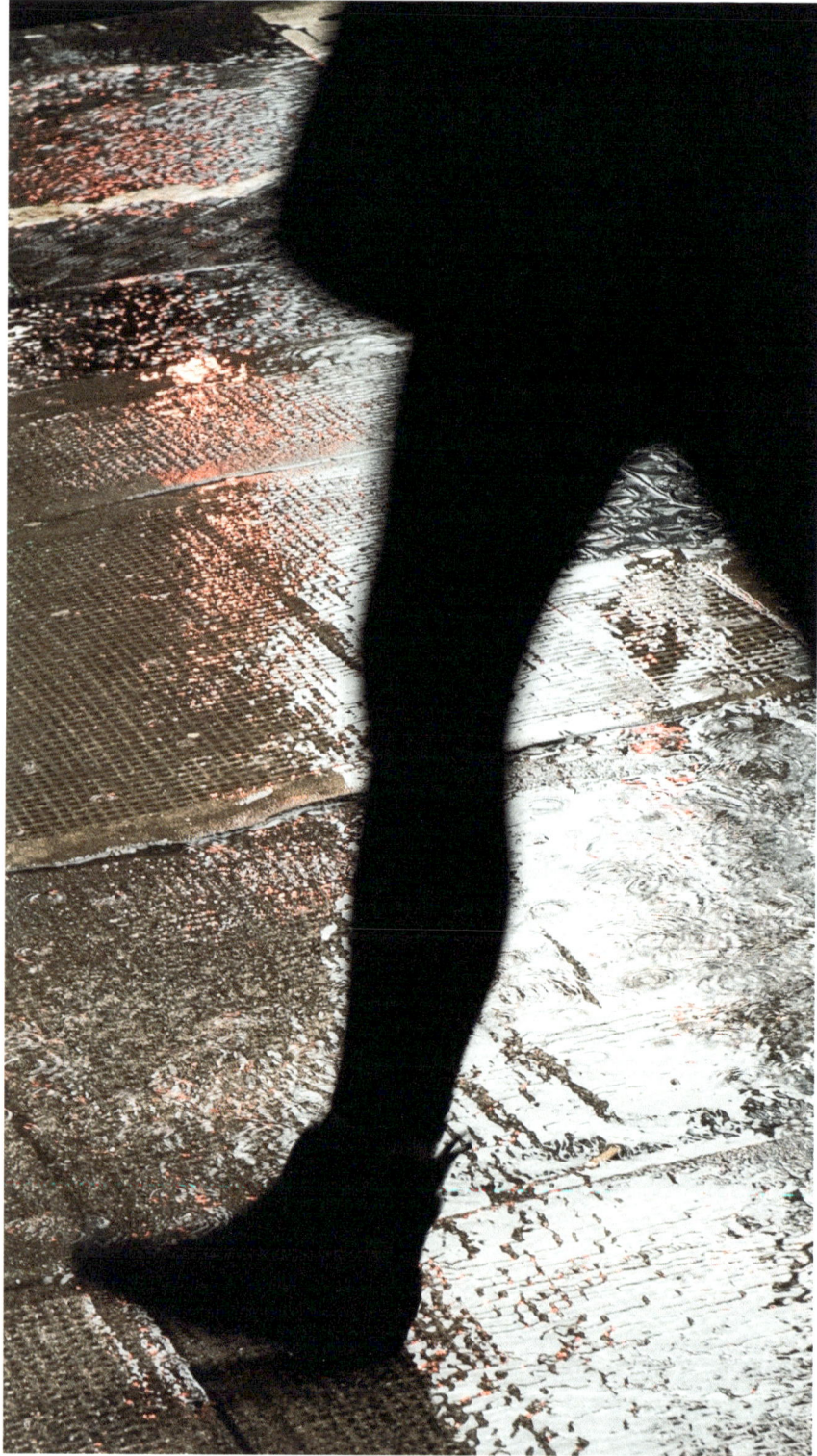

Day 17

PRAY FOR FOSTER KIDS, RUNAWAY CHILDREN, AND YOUTH

Father, my heart is continually shattered for what these children have walked through. The hand they were dealt was unfair. They've paid the price for someone else's mistakes and it's heavy. I've seen what it has done to their hearts, to their sense of security, to their trust of others, to their self worth, and it breaks me.

Lord, make Yourself known to these kids. May they find rest in You. May they find healing in You. May they see that their worth is not defined by what has happened to them, but in You and in You alone. May they be surrounded by a love so great, that they are able to choose different for themselves than the example set.

The industry looks like it has it all … love, support, family, a home. Often times things these kids feel they will never have. But Lord, I pray for Your protection over them when these lies come knocking. May they find refuge and freedom in You. Lord, I pray that You take away feelings of hopelessness and depression because these foster kids, runaway children, and youth are at a higher risk to be manipulated and falling victims to human trafficking. Father, release your anointing to heal their hurts and hearts. Amen.

The Lord is my shepherd, I lack nothing. He makes me lie down in green pastures, he leads me beside quiet waters, he refreshes my soul. He guides me along the right paths for his name's sake. Even though I walk through the darkest valley, I will fear no evil, for you are with me; your rod and your staff, they comfort me.

Psalm 23:1-4

OTHER SCRIPTURE VERSES TO READ

Psalm 12:5, Psalm 20:1, Psalm 46:1, Psalm 59:1, Psalm 140:4, Psalm 121

journal + notes

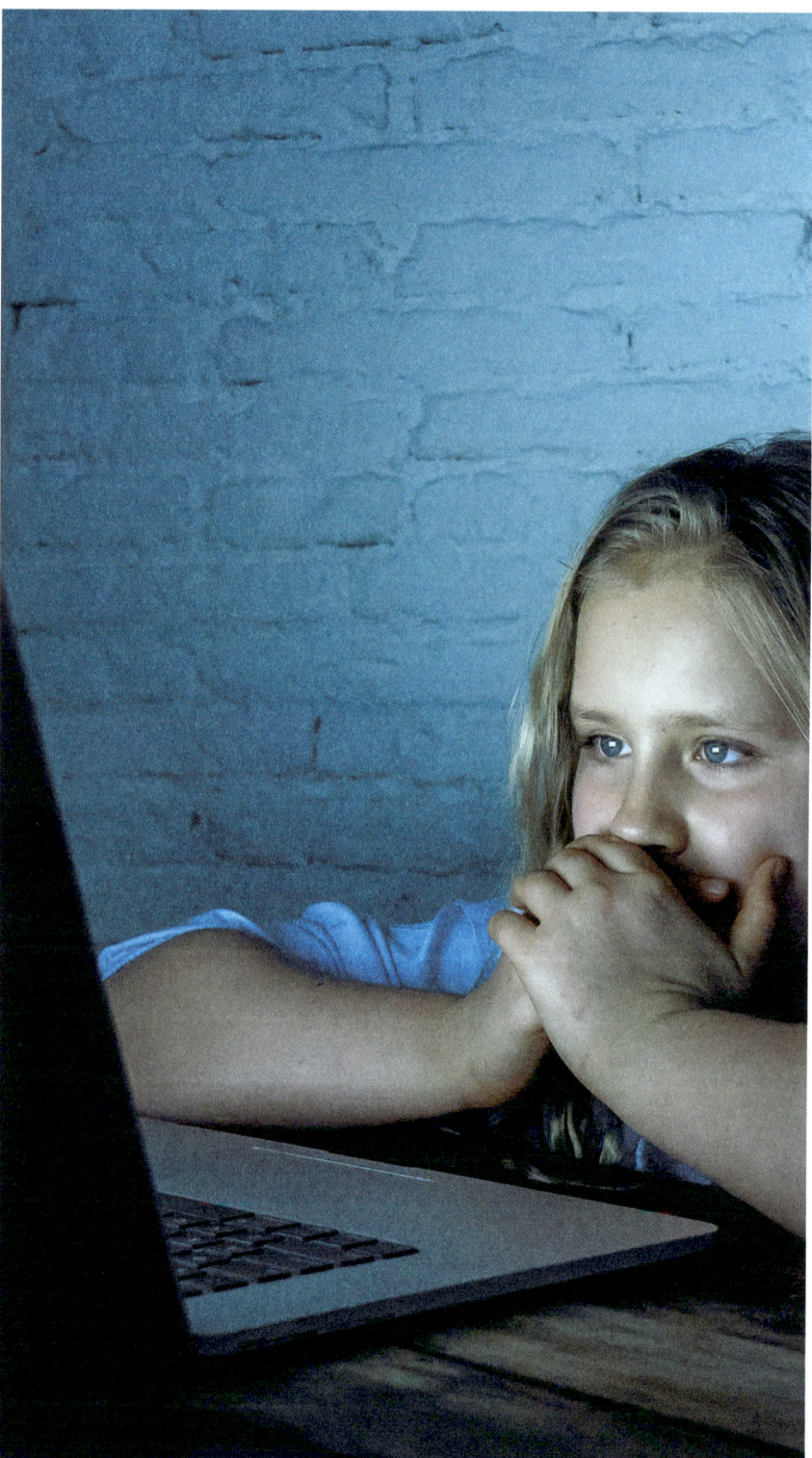

Day 18

PRAY FOR PREDATORS ON THE INTERNET AND SOCIAL MEDIA

Lord, I come today into the battle against the enemy who comes to steal, kill, and destroy. I pray for Your supernatural protection over those who are using the Internet and social media. As tools that were created to communicate and learn, they are now also being used to spread evil and sinful behaviors. You have given me the power and authority to bind, rebuke, and render powerless, the actions of perpetrators. Keep all of us safe from evil intention or persons of perversion and sexual immorality.

I pray for children and youth who are putting themselves at risk by communicating online with individuals they do not know. Individuals who are using entrapment tactics online to groom, befriend, establish emotional connections and relationships to gain their trust, romance them, control and manipulate their sexual curiosities, and lure them with deceitful actions to sexually exploit them. Lord, cover our children and youth with Your hedge of protection, and send Your angels to guard every one of them from this evil.

Lord, I also pray for people that are using the Internet and social media in ways that do not glorify You. I pray for those who are sinning, exposing themselves and others

Prayer continues on the next page.

Continued prayer from previous page.

to sexual immorality, pornography, and sextortion. I pray against the sexual obsessions and compulsions of pedophiles who are seeking child pornography. Bring to light the wicked hearts and deceitful actions of these sexual predators. Demolish the scales over the eyes of those addicted and ensnared by the binding power of pornography, that You can work a miracle in their lives. Let them not be taken captive by lust or their sexual fantasies, and preserve them from these sinful pleasures so that they can live beautiful lives away from this addiction.

There are millions of children and youth who are currently vulnerable to predators. I pray for those who have low self-esteem, have feelings of discouragement and unhealthy home environments, feel unworthy and hopeless, or feel that they have run out of options. Give them hope, worth, strength, and purpose. Equip them with a healthy identity that they are priceless and an unconditional worth. I pray today that You protect our children and youth from sexual abuses, sexually perverse criminals, predators, rapists, and sex traffickers who are using the Internet, apps, chat rooms, and social media to groom and arrange in-person meetings with their next victims. Lord, increase a Holy Spirit alarm in them from perpetrators so that our children and youth can flee from these dangers before they get trapped. Turn their hearts and minds towards You Lord. In Your name I pray, Amen.

journal + notes

What comes out of a person is what defiles them. For it is from within, out of a person's heart, that evil thoughts come—sexual immorality, theft, murder, adultery, greed, malice, deceit, lewdness, envy, slander, arrogance and folly. All these evils come from inside and defile a person.

Mark 7:20-23

OTHER SCRIPTURE VERSES TO READ

1 Corinthians 6:18, 1 Peter 5:8-9, Galatians 5:24, Philippians 4:8, Ephesians 5:3-4, Romans 12:2

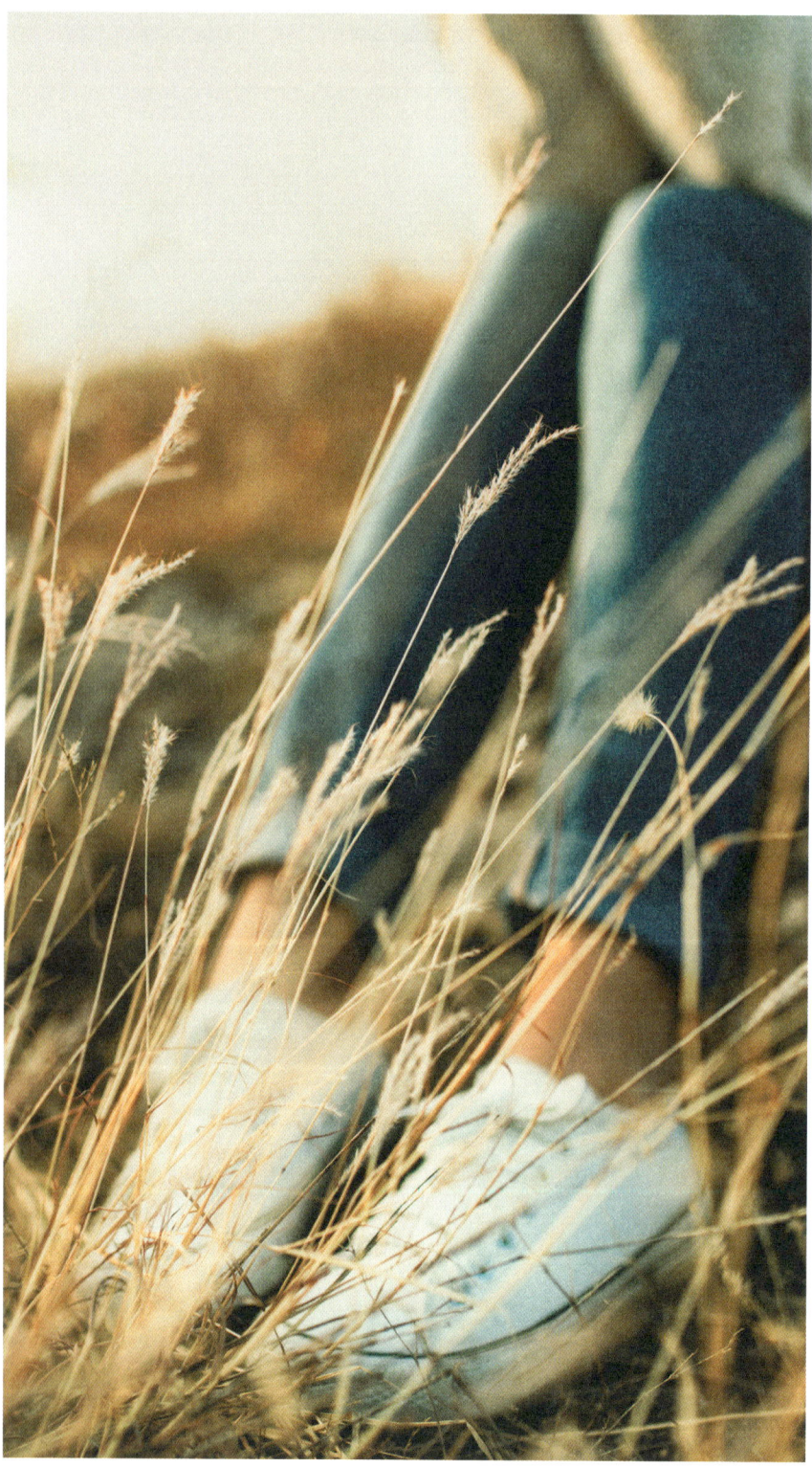

Day 19
PRAY FOR THOSE RECOVERING FROM TRAFFICKING TRAUMA

Dear Lord, thank You for freeing trafficking survivors from their horrific slavery. I know that You have come to this earth to set the captives free, and I am thankful that You are a God who saves. Today I ask special blessings over trafficking survivors who have been freed from the bondages of human trafficking and who are searching for healing. Father, their wounds are deep, their hurts are often unbearable, but I know that You have a plan and purpose for their life.

I ask today that each survivor would be put on a path that leads them to the safety, security, and stability that You desire for them. I pray today that each survivor would know unconditional love and that You would help them to regain their confidence in who they are, who You say they are, as a child of God. May You bring individuals into their life that will help to grow and sustain their relationship with You. God, You are amazing, and I am honored to be called Your child. Thank You for what You have done for those freed from trafficking, but most of all God, thank You for what You are going to do in the lives of those who are recovering from the trauma of trafficking. May You put a new song in their mouth as You raise them from the ashes, knowing that their testimony will reach others who have lived through the same trauma. In Your precious name, Amen

I waited patiently for the Lord; he turned to me and heard my cry. He lifted me out of the slimy pit, out of the mud and mire; he set my feet on a rock and gave me a firm place to stand. He put a new song in my mouth, a hymn of praise to our God. Many will see and fear the Lord and put their trust in him.

Psalm 40:1-3

OTHER SCRIPTURE VERSES TO READ

Genesis 50:20, Isaiah 40:31, Jeremiah 17:14, Jeremiah 30:17, 2 Corinthians 5:17, 1 Peter 5:7, Jeremiah 29:11 Ephesians 4:22-24, Psalm 51:10-12, Jeremiah 31:25, Matthew 11:29

journal + notes

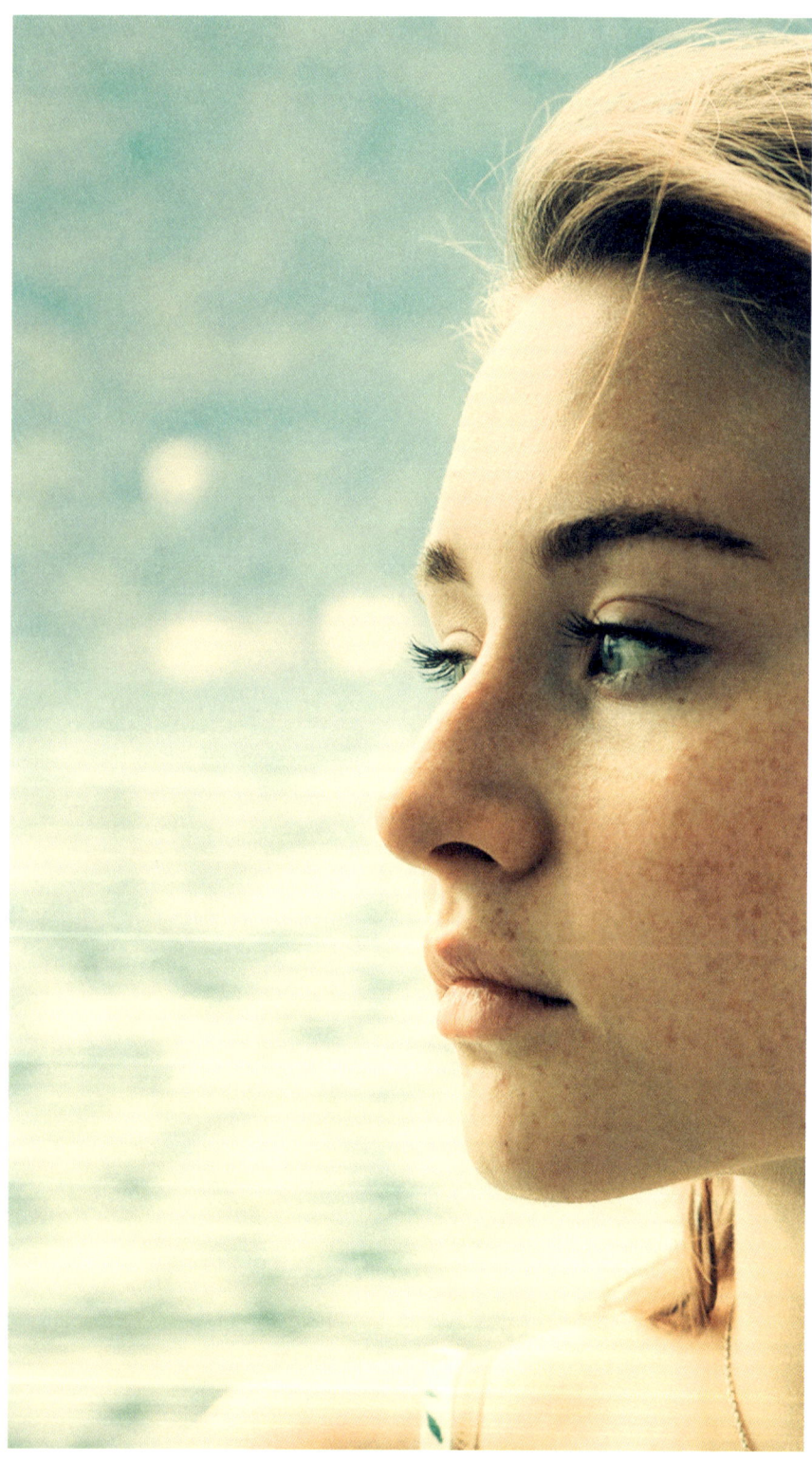

Day 20
PRAY FOR RESTORATION AND HEALING OF SURVIVORS PAST

Lord, I come to You in the name of Jesus, and I pray over these young women and men who are survivors of human trafficking. I pray over these young women and men who are seeking rehabilitation from domestic human trafficking. I pray today that they receive the long-term help needed to heal their mind, their body, and their spirit through holistic restoration. I pray for supernatural healing over their minds and that they know where their new identity lies.

Thank You Lord that survivors can transition into independent living and can discover their passions, explore career paths, and learn new skills for a chance at sustainability and independence. Your word says that they have the mind of Christ, and I pray that over these young women and men, that their minds are flooded with Your thoughts and Your Word. Lord, I know that You can only bring true freedom, and in the name of Jesus they are free from all bondages in their memories and in their hearts! You are the God of breakthrough, and I pray that over these young women and men right now. They are free. They are Yours. They have the mind of Christ. Satan has no jurisdiction on them any longer! In Jesus' name, Amen!

Forget the former things; do not dwell on the past. See, I am doing a new thing. Now it springs up; do you not perceive it? I am making a way in the wilderness and streams in the wasteland.

Isaiah 43:18-19

OTHER SCRIPTURE VERSES TO READ

Isaiah 43:25, 2 Corinthians 12:9-10, Romans 8:28, Romans 5:3-5, Ephesians 4:31-32

journal + notes

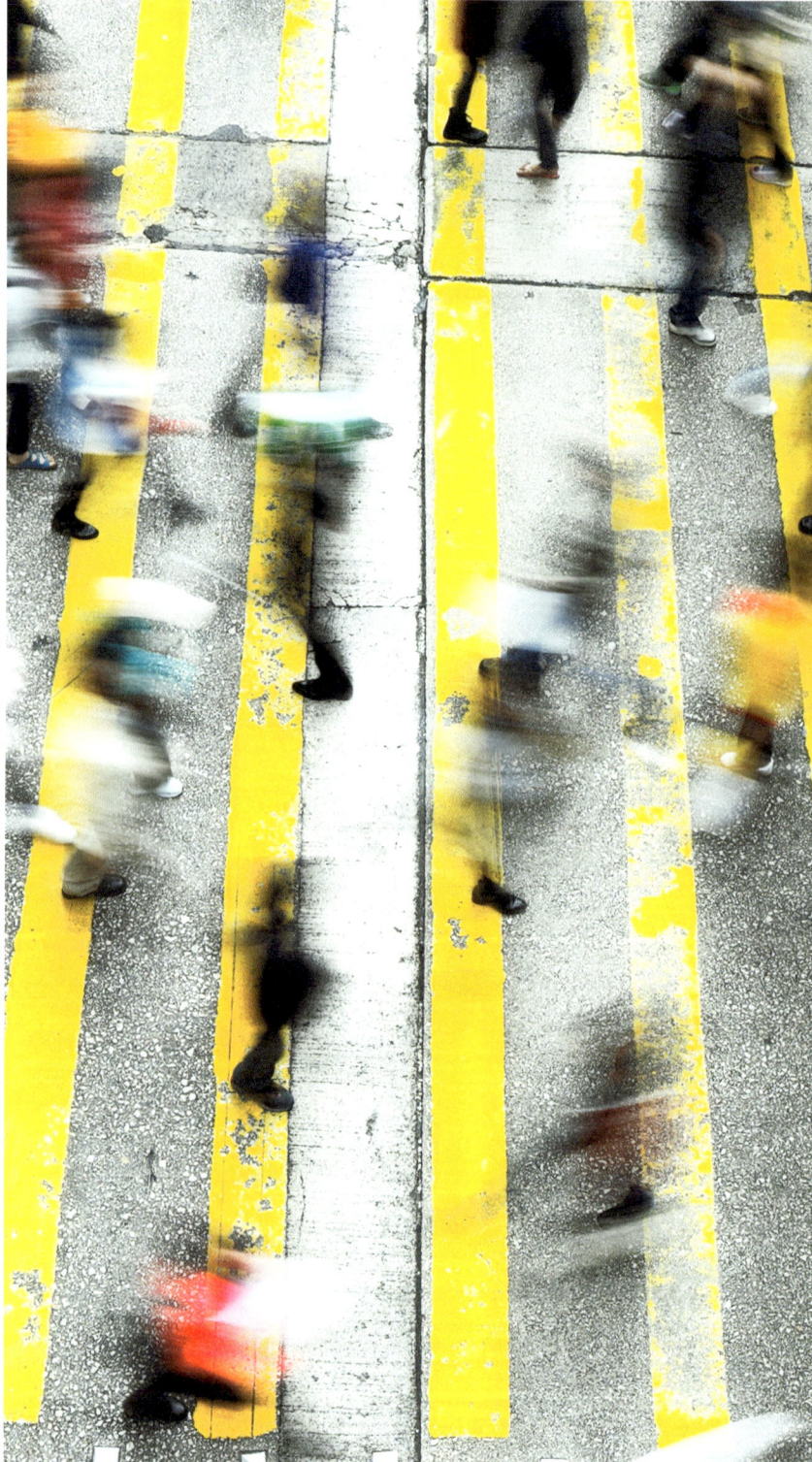

Day 21
PRAY FOR JUSTICE AND MERCY FOR TRAFFICKERS

Father of righteousness and mercy, I ask You for justice and mercy to come to those who traffic people. I ask for authorities to locate, arrest, prosecute, and sentence each one so that the unthinkable harm they are causing can no longer go forth. I ask for divine wisdom and discernment for the authorities who search for these traffickers and that Your justice will prevail.

Father, You sent Your Son to redeem us from our sin, but many have rejected Your plan and turned from the abundant life that it is in Jesus Christ. I pray for all who are responsible for the unthinkable crime of human trafficking, and that Your power would break through resulting in salvation and a new life in Christ. I pray for a restorative justice, which brings about true healing and forgiveness for both human trafficking victims and the offender. As Jesus' saving grace enters into places of depravity, I pray for radically changed hearts, complete freedom, and for powerful testimonies of transformed lives for Christ. May the Heavens shake with praise as God breaks through to the most hardened criminal and to those who have suffered at their hand. Amen

Who executes justice for the oppressed, who gives food to the hungry. The Lord sets the prisoners free.

Psalm 146:7

OTHER SCRIPTURE VERSES TO READ

Psalm 103:6, Psalm 37:17, Isaiah 16:4, Jeremiah 22:3, Amos 5:15a, 1 Timothy 6:10a

journal + notes

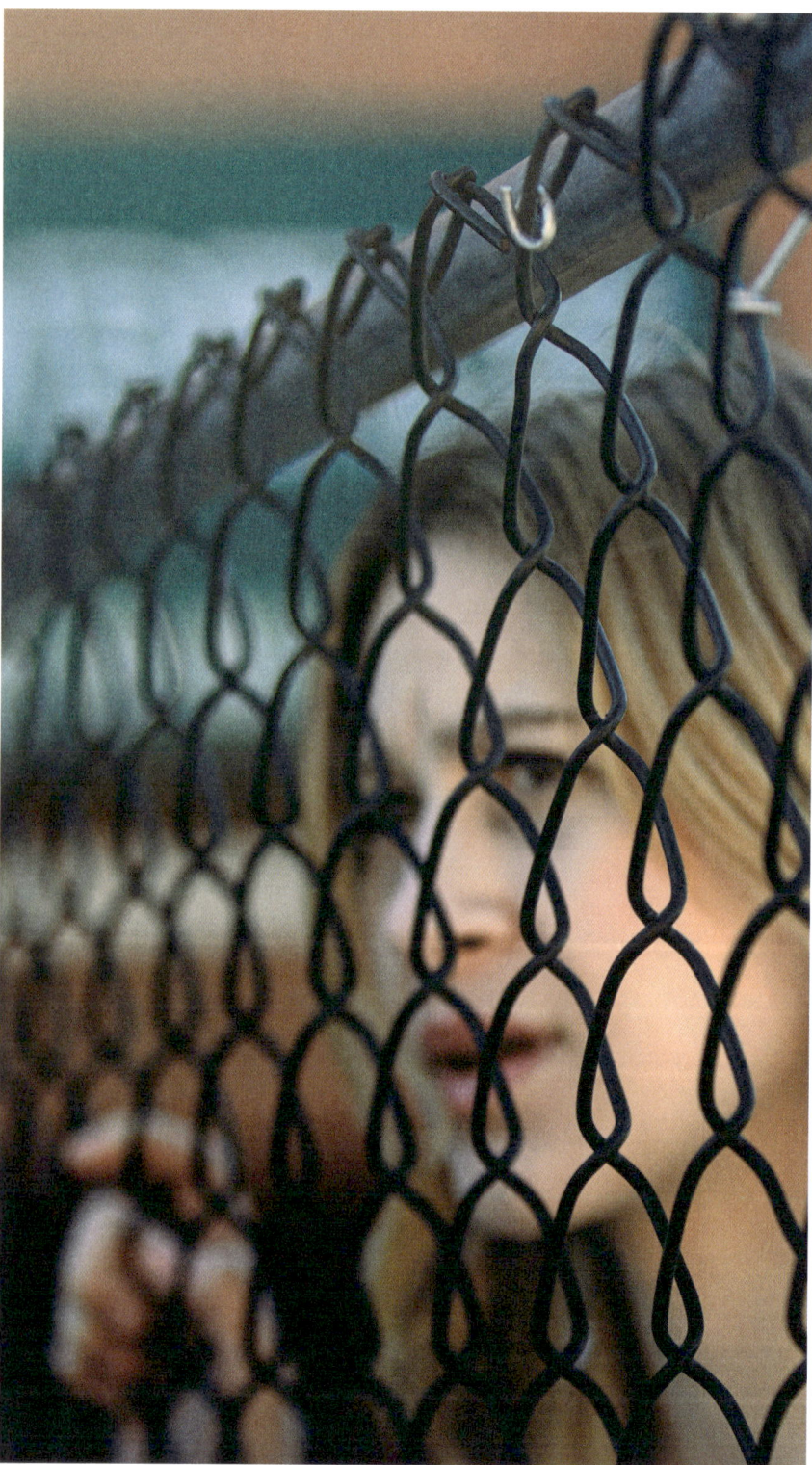

Day 22
PRAY FOR GOD TO DISMANTLE TRAFFICKING RINGS

Heavenly Father, I boldly come before Your throne to pray for the dismantling of trafficking rings and bind them in Jesus' name. I pray that Your light would uncover hidden schemes and networks of those managing these rings. I pray for wisdom, discernment, and courage for law enforcement as they work to uncover and arrest those involved. I pray that You would bring confusion into the enemy's camp so that his schemes are thwarted, that they are unorganized and ineffective.

I thank You Jesus that You came to the earth to save sinners. All of us have sinned and fallen short, but You love us anyway, yes even those who seek to enslave others. I have read in Your Word of people like the Apostle Paul who once persecuted Christians but were changed in a moment by an encounter with You. I pray that Your Spirit would encounter these perpetrators in miraculous ways to convict their hearts of the reality of what they are doing and that they would not only seek help, but that they would repent and accept Your free gift of salvation. I thank You God for Your love for us and declare that through You that nothing is impossible! Amen.

But the Lord your God will deliver them over to you, throwing them into great confusion until they are destroyed.

Deuteronomy 7:23

OTHER SCRIPTURE VERSES TO READ

Psalm 71:24, Isaiah 55:7, Romans 5:6-8, Psalm 7:9, Psalm 37:17

journal + notes

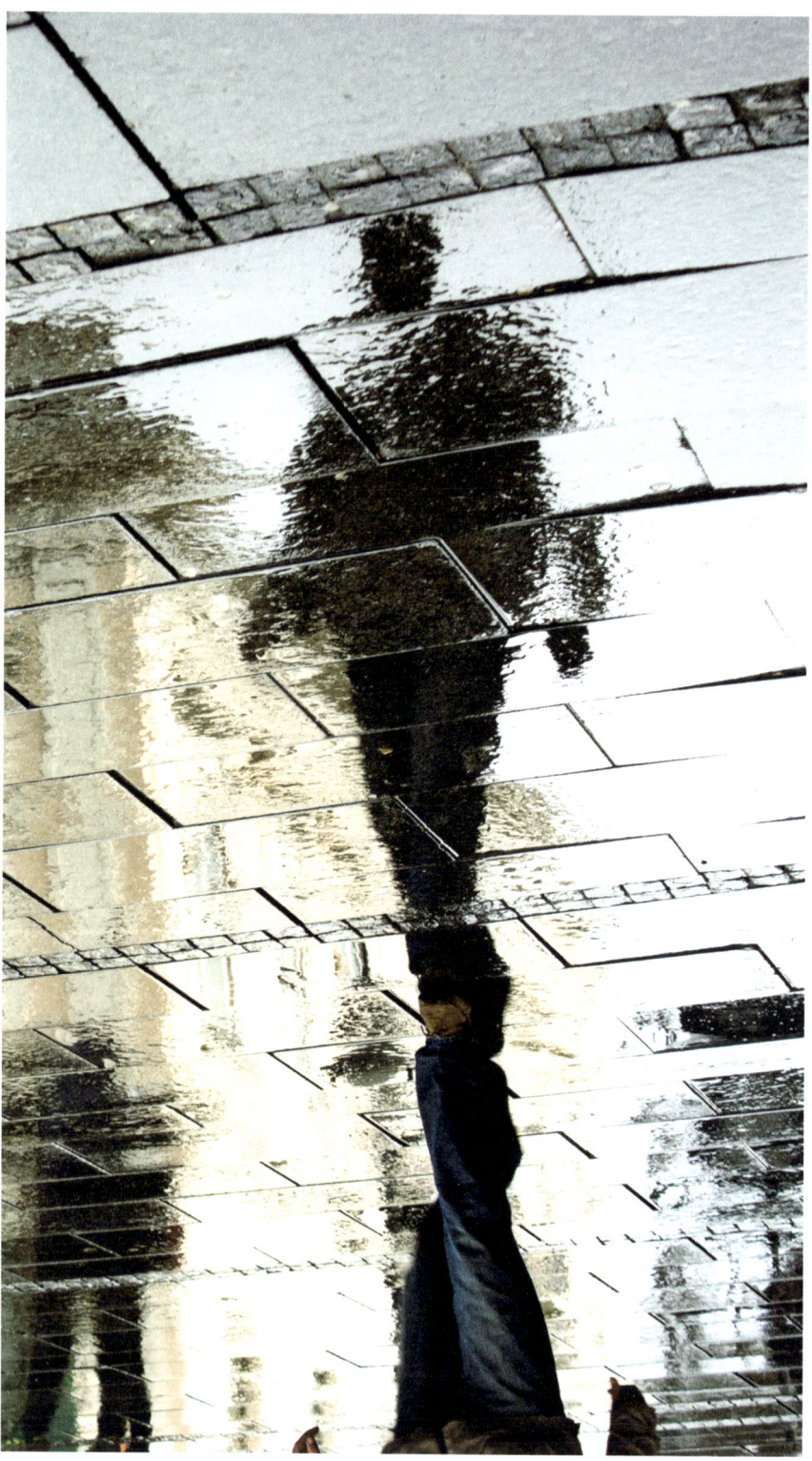

Day 23

PRAY FOR BUYERS (JOHNS*)

*"Johns" is a term used for customers (predominantly men) who seek to solicit and purchase sex or sexual entertainment from traffickers/pimps.

Lord Jesus, I pray for the "Johns" who are overwhelmed by selfishness, lust, and greed. I pray for the end of pornography, prostitution, and strip clubs. I pray that commercial sex trafficking would cease to exist. I ask, Holy Spirit, that You would remove the sin that blinds these "Johns," and open their eyes to the evil and destructive behavior they commit.

Lord Jesus, I also pray that You would move in our hearts for these "Johns" who are enslaved to this evil. I pray that I would not see them as just customers or consumers who seek to solicit and purchase sex, but that I see these "Johns" as You see them, made in Your image, but ravaged with sin, broken, and lost from their original design that can only be found in You.

As I pray and declare that You will set the captive free, as Your children, I cry out and pray for our brothers and sisters enslaved in exploiting others through this sin of sex trafficking. Holy Spirit, stir in the broken hearts of these "Johns" and help them realize the same forgiveness and salvation that was extended to the thief

Prayer continues on the next page.

Continued prayer from previous page.

on the cross, can be extended to them. Help these "Johns" to realize that it is never too late to turn to You - Jesus! I pray this in the powerful and wonderful name of Jesus!

In his arrogance the wicked man hunts down the weak, who are caught in the schemes he devises. He boasts about the cravings of his heart; he blesses the greedy and reviles the Lord. In his pride the wicked man does not seek him; in all his thoughts there is no room for God. He lies in wait near the villages; from ambush he murders the innocent. His eyes watch in secret for his victims; like a lion in cover he lies in wait. He lies in wait to catch the helpless; he catches the helpless and drags them off in his net. His victims are crushed, they collapse; they fall under his strength. He says to himself, "God will never notice; he covers his face and never sees."

Psalm 10:2-4; 8-11

OTHER SCRIPTURE VERSES TO READ

Matthew 5:44, Leviticus 19:29, Joel 3:3-6, Luke 12:15, Psalm 34:17-20

journal + notes

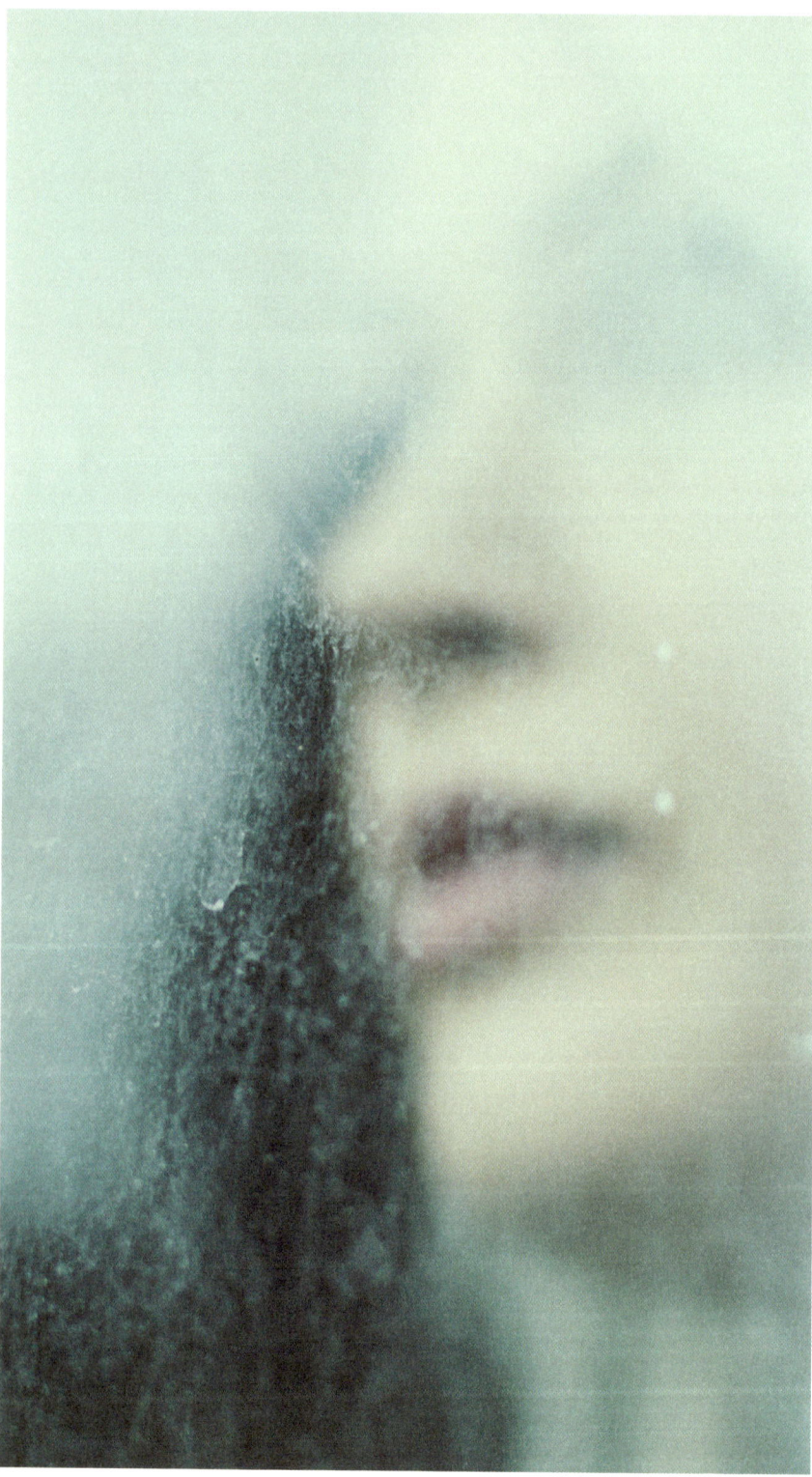

Day 24
PRAY FOR ABUSERS AND PERPETRATORS

Dear Heavenly Father, in 1 John 3:1-2 You remind us that we are Your beloved children, even if we are not recognized as such by the world. You say that although it is not yet apparent to the visible world what we will become, You see our potential! I pray that abusers and perpetrators of human trafficking will know that they are also children of God! I pray for forgiveness for them, Lord. I pray that I may be willing to forgive them. I pray that You teach them Your truth: that they are never too lost to be forgiven.

I plead the blood of Jesus for healing inside and out for their hearts and minds. I pray that You would help the world become willing to see the abuser and perpetrator the way that You see them; as Your child. Purify their minds and obsessions. Take away their thoughts and urges so they stop relying on themselves and start to fully trust in You, Lord.

I pray that society will become willing to recognize that empathy for the perpetrator does not come at the expense of the victim. A perpetrator is usually a victim wearing a different colored cloak. This is why You told Peter to forgive 7x70 times! Because forgiveness of self and others is essential. In Jesus' precious name, Amen.

But I tell you, love your enemies and pray for those who persecute you, that you may be children of your Father in heaven. He causes his sun to rise on the evil and the good, and sends rain on the righteous and the unrighteous.

Matthew 5:44-45

OTHER SCRIPTURE VERSES TO READ

1 John 3:1-2 , Ephesians 4:32, Luke 6:27, Luke 6:37, Mark 11:25, 1 Peter 3:8-4:19, 1 Peter 1:13

journal + notes

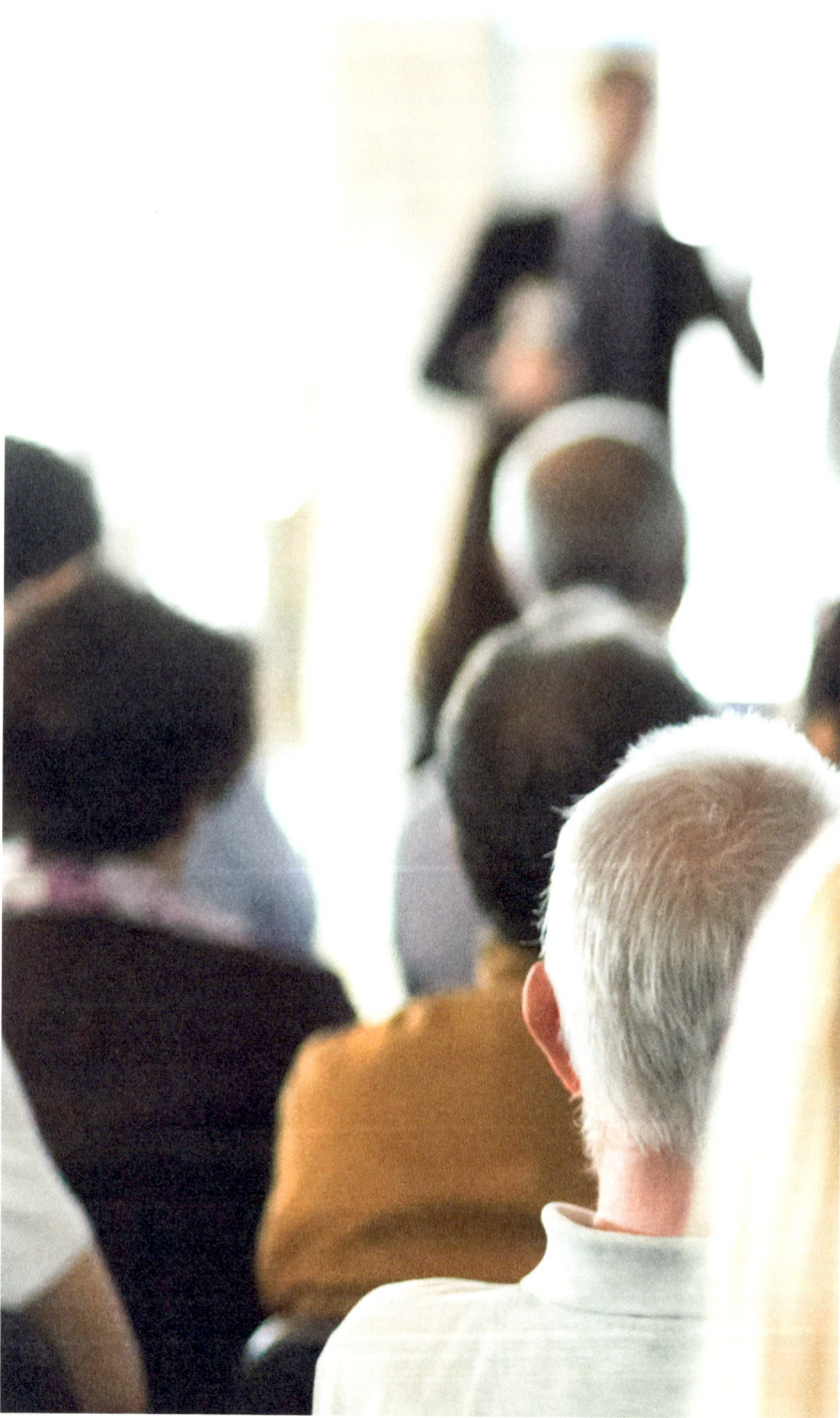

Day 25
PRAY FOR GOVERNMENT LEADERS

Heavenly Father, I thank You for the leaders you have placed over us. I pray that You will bless them for their willingness to serve in my community, state, and nation. I ask for Your protection over our leaders and their families. May they feel Your love, mercy, and encouragement and I ask that You strengthen them when they are weary.

Thank You especially for those that have stood with the anti-trafficking movement to protect the most vulnerable in our communities. Help them to have the humility to work with others to accomplish this task, and soften the hearts of more of our leaders to join this fight. Fill them with wisdom and knowledge to be able to strategize and enact the best methods to legislate change that will help in the fight to free these captives from sexual exploitation, trafficking, and abuse.

I also pray that You do not allow our leaders to fall into corruption but to always be trustworthy and committed to work for justice. Pour out Your spirit upon them and make Your Word known to them. Help them to be men and women of integrity with an understanding of Your principles, acting justly, and righteously. Bless them in Jesus' name, Amen.

I urge, then, first of all, that petitions, prayers, intercession and thanksgiving be made for all people—for kings and all those in authority, that we may live peaceful and quiet lives in all godliness and holiness.

1 Timothy 2:1-2

OTHER SCRIPTURE VERSES TO READ

Proverbs 8:15, Nehemiah 9:13, 1 Kings 3:12, Deuteronomy 16:19, Proverbs 3:21

journal + notes

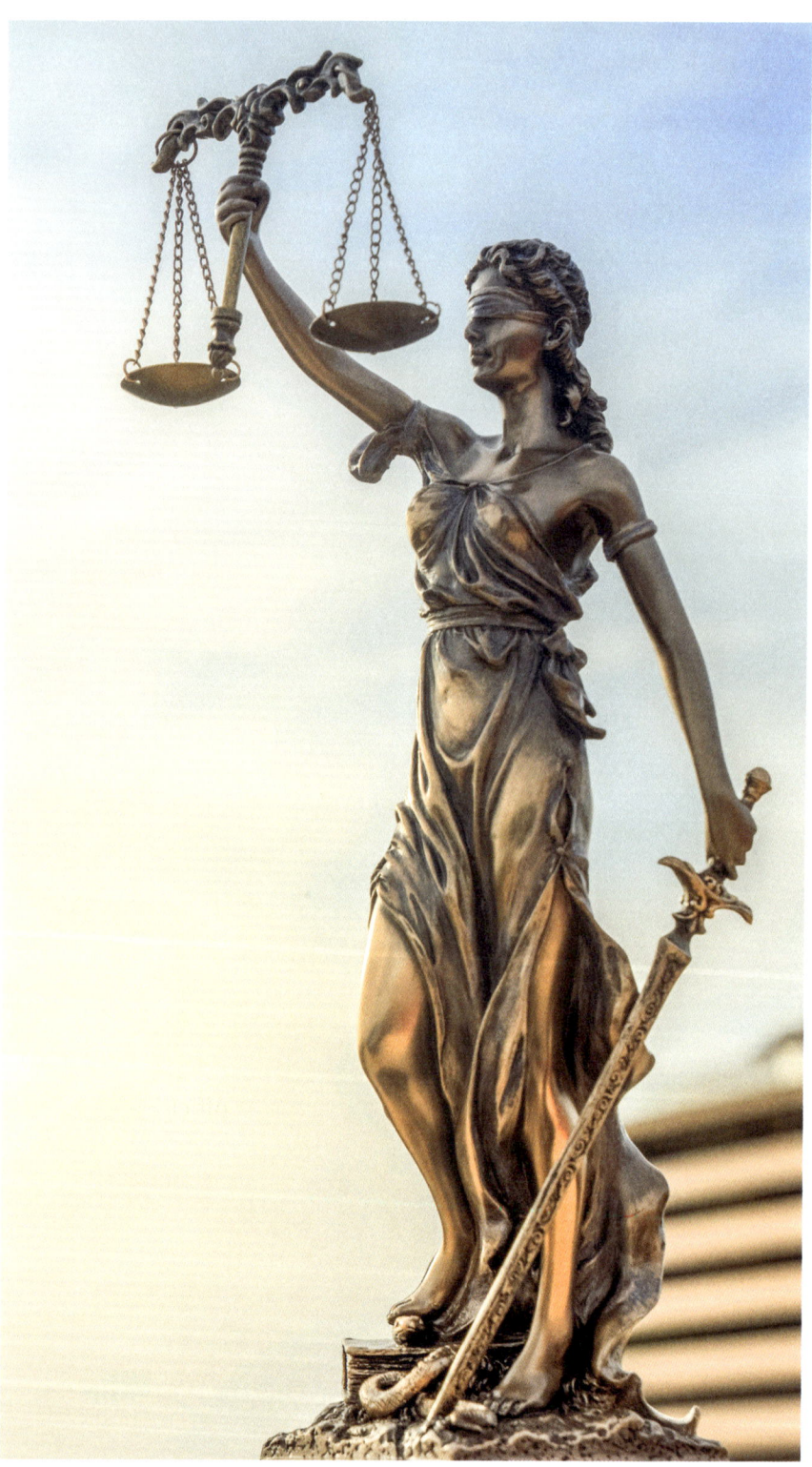

Day 26
PRAY FOR GOD HONORING LAWS OUTLAWING EXPLOITATION

God, I praise You for every single life on this earth and say that each life has incredible value because each is Your creation, made in Your image.

I ask for You to bring the faces and personal stories of human trafficking into every world leader's mind and heart. I ask You, Holy Spirit, to speak to world leaders with tremendous personal conviction affecting action to fight this injustice.

I speak against every level of corruption in government and law enforcement, from local to national levels. I pray for governments to stand on the side of the victims and that every government worker and law official to have awareness of trafficking in their area so they can implement appropriate, just legislation outlawing the exploitation of people.

I pray for new legislation to prevent the buying and selling of products made from slaves and illegal markets fueled by slave labor. I ask that these laws

Prayer continues on the next page.

Continued prayer from previous page.

would prosecute and bring appropriate justice to the traffickers and purchasers.

I pray for wisdom and understanding for law enforcement and law makers—that the implementation of laws and creation of laws would be fully informed about the issues of trafficking. Lord, I pray for human trafficking and the enslavement of Your sons and daughters to come to an end, through raising up leaders in government and creation of laws. In Jesus' name, Amen.

Therefore, you kings, be wise; be warned, you rulers of the earth. Serve the Lord with fear and celebrate his rule with trembling.

Psalms 2:10-11

OTHER SCRIPTURE VERSES TO READ

Isaiah 10:1-2, Deuteronomy 16:19, Proverbs 8:15, 1 Kings 3:12

journal + notes

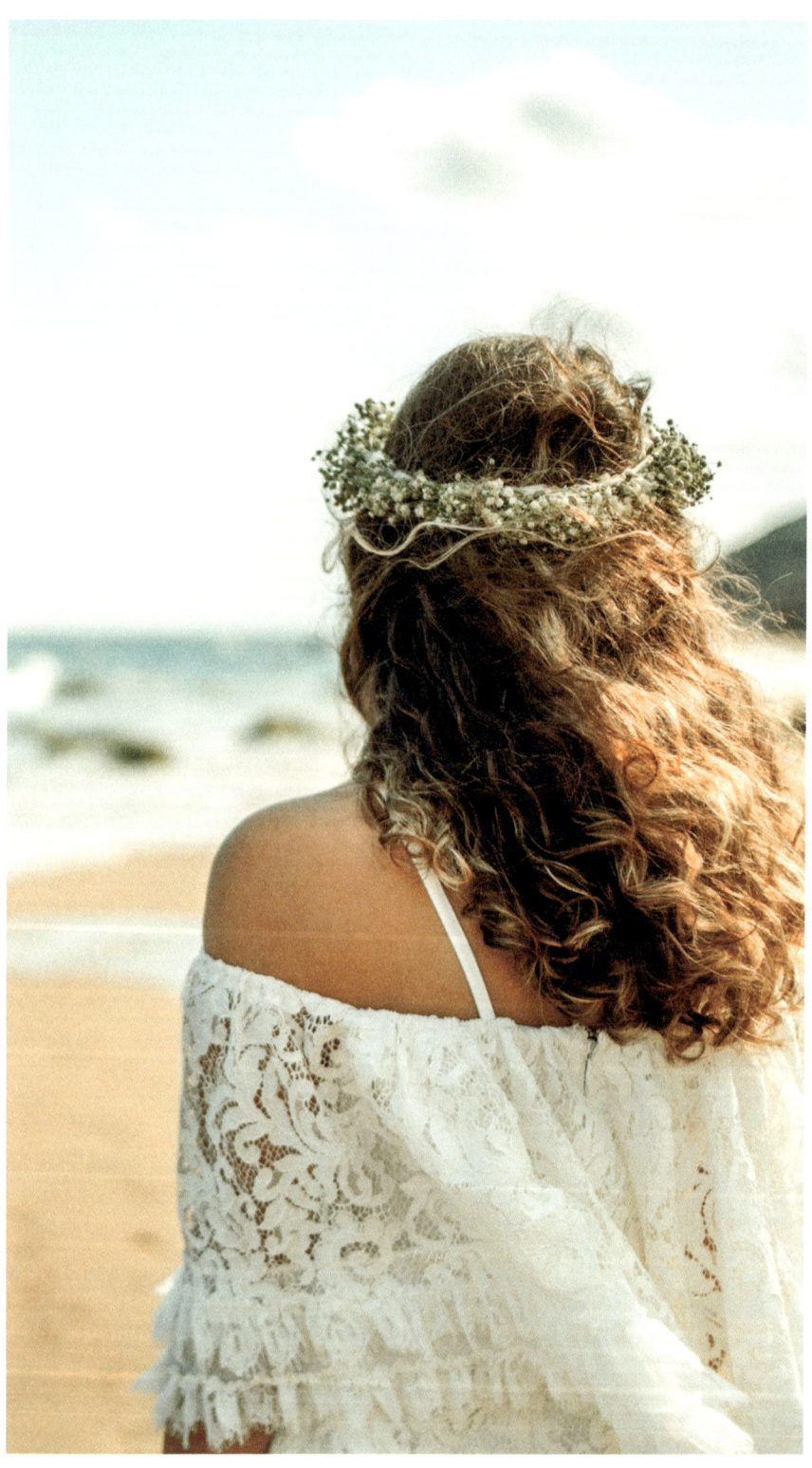

Day 27
PRAY FOR THE CHURCH TO AWAKEN AND RISE UP TO THE ISSUE

Lord God, I come before You with a sincere heart. With gratefulness and thanks that You would hear my prayers. Father, please open the eyes of church leaders and their congregations to the truth of what is happening in this world regarding human trafficking. Father, I pray that their eyes would see the truth and stir their hearts with compassion for these people, for they are fearfully and wonderfully made in Your image. Lord, I pray that You stir their hearts to take action on behalf of these dear souls.

I pray for church leaders and interested people of faith to prayerfully consider how to collaborate for awareness, prevention, and intervention in their communities and cities. Lord I pray for churches to rise up and support nonprofits and other organizations on the frontlines so they can be the hands and feet of help. Give the church eyes to see and ears to hear so they may reach out to those who are being victimized and in bondage of modern-day slavery. Please Father, protect these victims from harm. Give them strength to stand as the church embraces them with love and care. I pray this in the mighty name of Jesus, Amen.

Who will rise up for me against the wicked? Who will take a stand for me against evildoers?

Psalms 94:16

OTHER SCRIPTURE VERSES TO READ

Proverbs 31:8, Matthew 5:13-14, Matthew 9:37-38, Matthew 16:18, Psalm 133

journal + notes

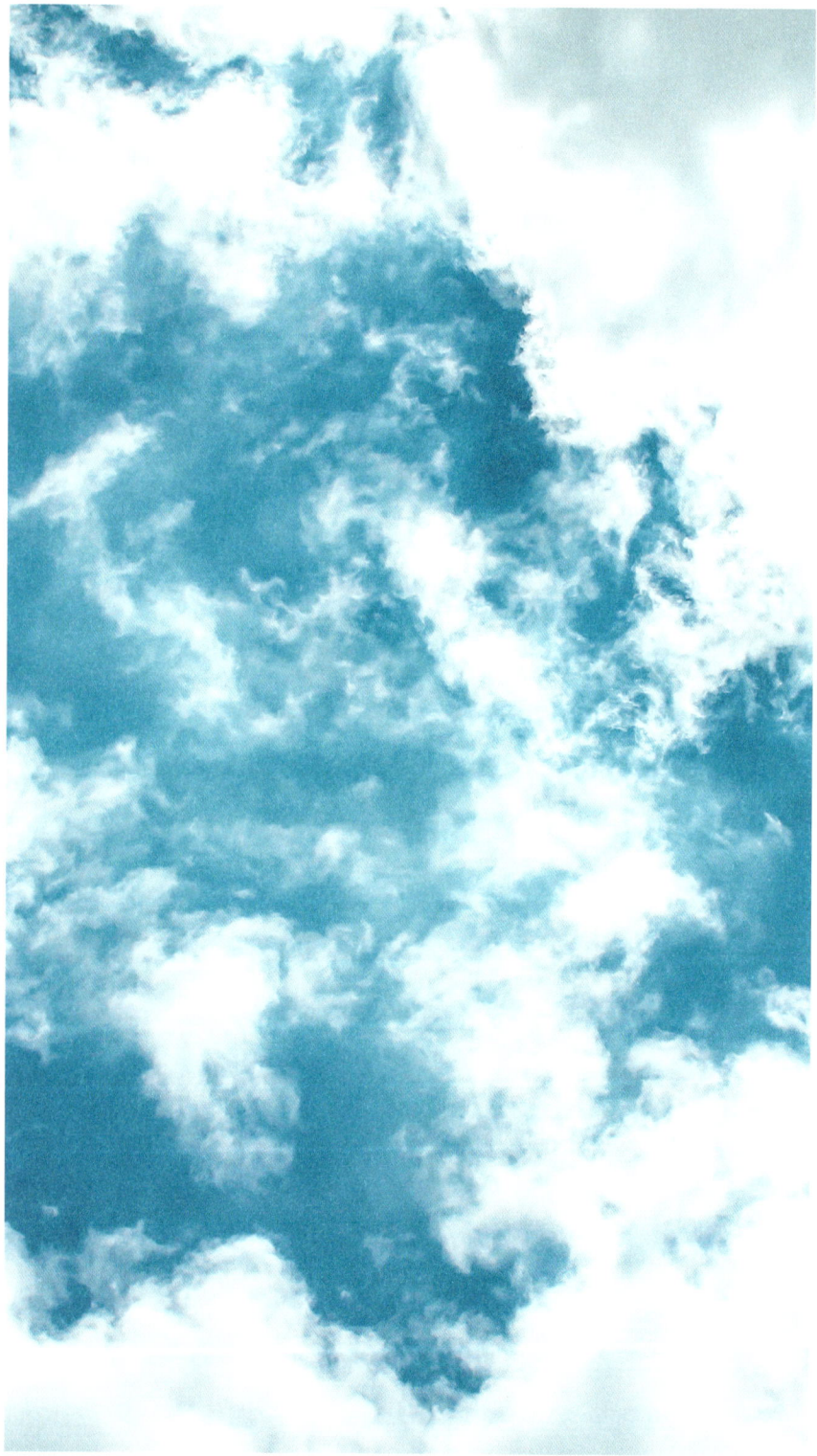

Day 28
PRAY FOR THE CHURCH, ITS MEMBERS AND LEADERS

Heavenly Father, today, I pray for Your church to rise up and speak for the helpless, vulnerable, imprisoned, and oppressed. I ask that You awaken the issue of modern-day slavery in our churches across our country and bring unity between denominations so that all of us can unite to end this evil.

Father, I pray for church members and church leaders to remain sexually pure and that they not become the perpetrators or consumers of abuse in any form. I pray for new laborers to come out of the church for this cause.

Father, I pray for Your church to be the top defender of our children and protector of our communities. I pray that the people of Your church are willing to work and pray daily to bring an end to human trafficking and sexual exploitation. In Jesus' name I pray, Amen!

The Spirit of the Sovereign Lord is on me, because the Lord has anointed me to proclaim good news to the poor. He has sent me to bind up the brokenhearted, to proclaim freedom for the captives and release from darkness for the prisoners, to proclaim the year of the Lord's favor and the day of vengeance of our God, to comfort all who mourn, and provide for those who grieve in Zion—to bestow on them a crown of beauty instead of ashes, the oil of joy instead of mourning, and a garment of praise instead of a spirit of despair. They will be called oaks of righteousness, a planting of the Lord for the display of his splendor.

Isaiah 61:1-3

OTHER SCRIPTURE VERSES TO READ

1 Peter 2:9-10, 1 Thessalonians 4:3-5, Proverbs 31:8
Ephesians 4:19-20

journal + notes

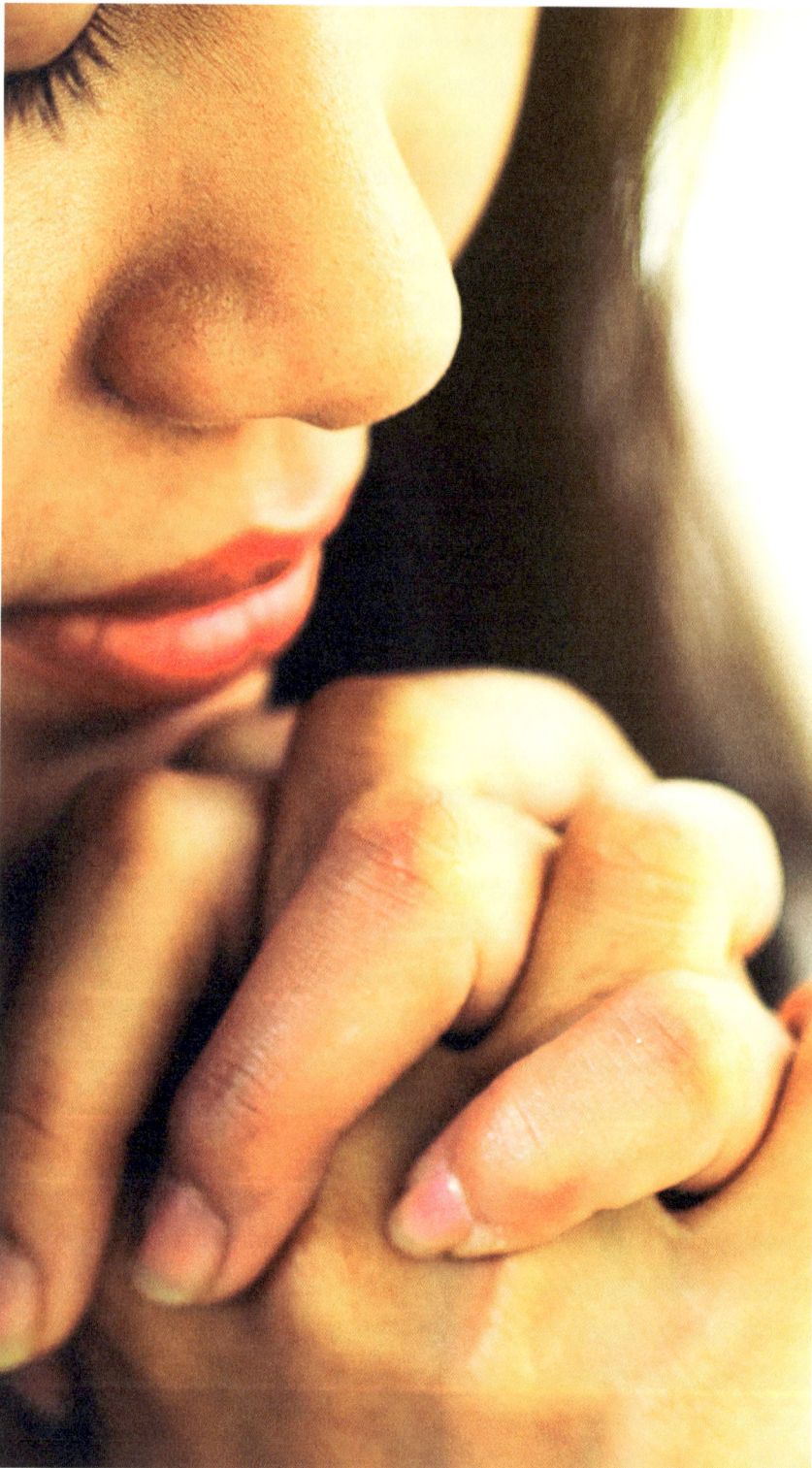

Day 29
PRAY FOR SALVATION OF TRAFFICKERS, BUYERS, AND VICTIMS

Heavenly Father, I pray for the men and women who are trafficking and purchasing individuals for their own pleasure and gain. I pray that they would hear Your voice loud and clear that what they are doing is wrong and that they would turn from their evil ways as they call on You seeking repentance and receiving Your gift of salvation through Your son, Jesus. I pray that they would join in the fight against sex trafficking and that they would become passionate advocates for social justice.

Father, I pray for the women, men, and children on the streets and in the hotels and homes who are being trafficked and exploited. I pray that they would sense Your presence even in their darkest times and know that You are with them, that You are for them, and that You love them. I pray that they would be directed to a safe place where they could seek the help they need and that their lives would be restored.

I pray that they would invite Your son, Jesus, to be their personal Savior and that they would then be warriors for You reaching others who are lost. I ask all of this in Jesus' name, Amen!

For the Son of Man came to seek and to save the lost.

Luke 19:10

OTHER SCRIPTURE VERSES TO READ

Matthew 5:43-47, Luke 6:27, Ephesians 4:32, John 3:16-17, Romans 5:8

journal + notes

31 DAYS OF PRAYER FOR HUMAN TRAFFICKING

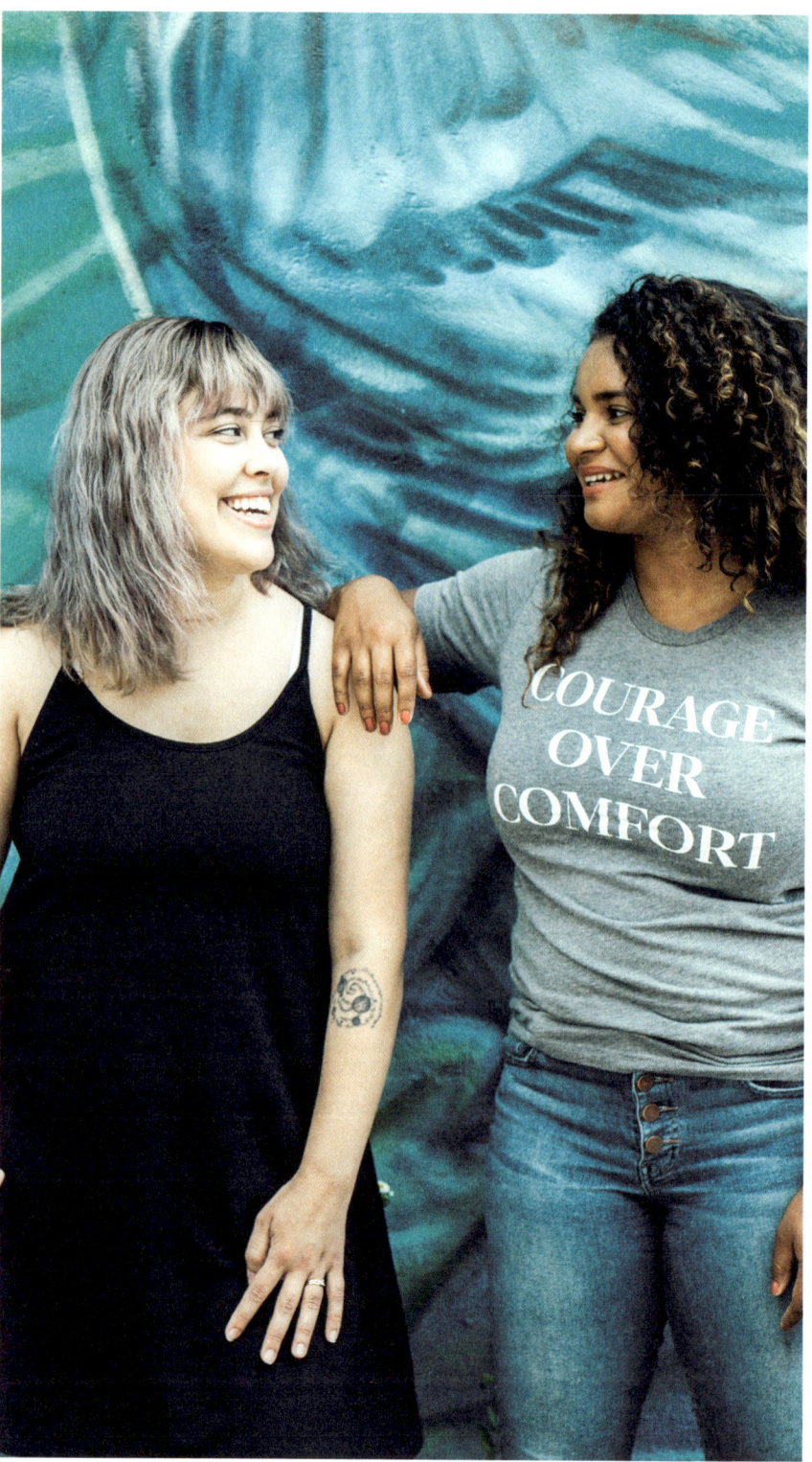

Day 30
PRAY FOR MINISTRIES AND ORGANIZATIONS FIGHTING TRAFFICKING

Abba Father, I come before You today to intercede on behalf of ministries and organizations combating human trafficking. I pray for those in leadership. Give them the strength to continue the fight. Do not let them be discouraged. Inspire them to use the talents and gifts You have blessed them with to further Your kingdom in unique and creative ways. May You guard their hearts from bitterness and fatigue. Protect their mental health as the exhaustion of the magnitude of their work weighs heavy.

Lord, when they are not sure where provision to continue on comes from, be their provision. When they aren't sure how they can move forward or when the road blocks of culture, money, and government, stand in their way, I know You can, and You will make a way. When there is outreach and awareness, Father, let those who need this message have open ears and softened hearts. You are the provider, the One who gives, who hears my prayers and answers them. Today I believe in Your power to fulfill Your promises. In Jesus' name, Amen.

Behold, I will do a new thing; now it shall spring forth; shall ye not know it? I will even make a way in the wilderness, and rivers in the desert.

Isaiah 43:91

OTHER SCRIPTURE VERSES TO READ

Psalm 90:17, Psalm 12:7-8, Psalm 34:15-18, Psalm 77:14, Isaiah 66:2, Proverbs 16:16

journal + notes

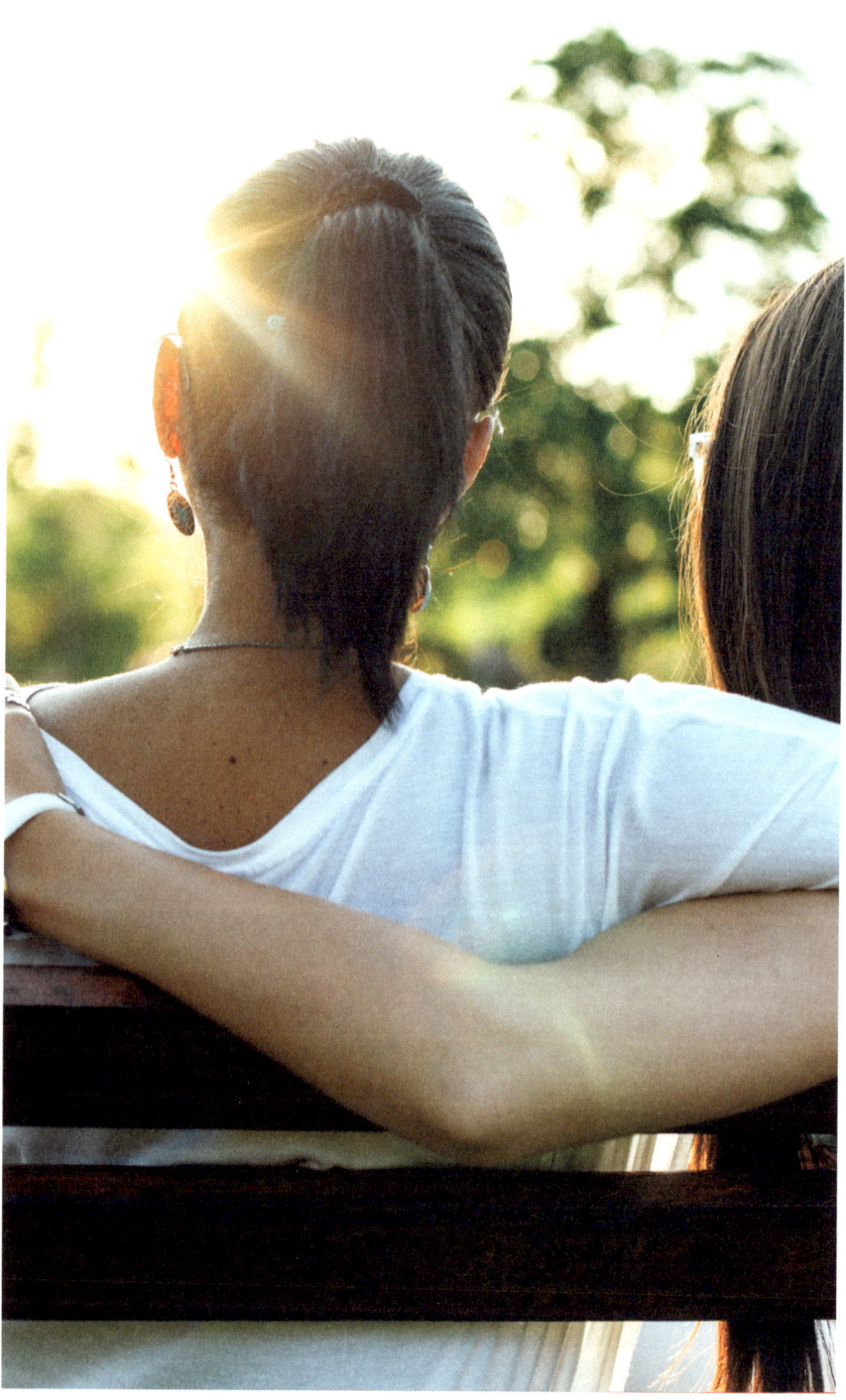

Day 31
PRAY FOR RESTORATION HOMES AND SAFE HOUSES

Jesus, I thank You for being the father of freedom and restoration. I am so grateful for the hope You provide when it feels like darkness is all around. Lord, You know the dire need we're facing for housing in our cities, state, and nation for victims of human trafficking.

I pray for Your strength and direction as individuals and organizations respond to the call You've put on their hearts to support or launch a restoration home. I ask that You cover those teams in Your blessing and protection, and that You draw them together as they work to bring freedom to those trapped in slavery. Fill their hearts with love and compassion for the survivors they will be serving, and guide their steps as they build new programs.

I pray that every home would be a beacon of hope for survivors. That every individual brought into these programs would find healing, restoration, and freedom in You. I pray new beginnings for survivors, living no longer as victims, but as victors. Use me, and raise up others, to abolish slavery. In Your name I pray, Amen.

Come to me, all you who are weary and burdened, and I will give you rest.

Matthew 11:28

OTHER SCRIPTURE VERSES TO READ

Matthew 25:34-40, Isaiah 61:1-3, Psalm 9:18, Hebrews 13:16, 2 Corinthians 5:17

journal + notes

Thank you for choosing this resource from Hope Inspire Love.

TOGETHER, WE ARE ERADICATING HUMAN TRAFFICKING AND SEXUAL EXPLOITATION IN OUR LIFETIME.

Freedom starts with **YOU**

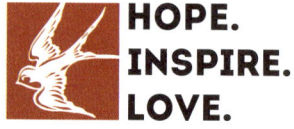

**HOPE.
INSPIRE.
LOVE.**

HOPEINSPIRELOVE.ORG/PRAY